Health as a Virtue

Princeton Theological Monograph Series

K. C. Hanson, Charles M. Collier, D. Christopher Spinks,
and Robin Parry, Series Editors

Recent volumes in the series:

Anette I. Hagan
*Eternal Blessedness for All? A Historical-Systematic Examination
of Schleiermacher's Understanding of Predestination*

Stephen M. Garrett
God's Beauty-in-Act: Participating in God's Suffering Glory

Sarah Morice-Brubaker
The Place of the Spirit: Toward a Trinitarian Theology of Location

Joas Adiprasetya
*An Imaginative Glimpse:
The Trinity and Multiple Religious Participations*

Anthony G. Siegrist
*Participating Witness: An Anabaptist Theology of Baptism
and the Sacramental Character of the Church*

Kin Yip Louie
*The Beauty of the Triune God:
The Theological Aesthetics of Jonathan Edwards*

Mark R. Lindsay
*Reading Auschwitz with Barth:
The Holocaust as Problem and Promise for Barthian Theology*

Brendan Thomas Sammon
*The God Who Is Beauty: Beauty as a Divine Name
in Thomas Aquinas and Dionysius the Areopagite*

Health as a Virtue

Thomas Aquinas and the Practice of Habits of Health

MELANIE L. DOBSON

☙PICKWICK *Publications* • Eugene, Oregon

HEALTH AS A VIRTUE
Thomas Aquinas and the Practice of Habits of Health

Princeton Theological Monograph Series 209

Copyright © 2014 Melanie L. Dobson. All rights reserved. Except for brief quotations in critical publications or reviews, no part of this book may be reproduced in any manner without prior written permission from the publisher. Write: Permissions, Wipf and Stock Publishers, 199 W. 8th Ave., Suite 3, Eugene, OR 97401.

Pickwick Publications
An Imprint of Wipf and Stock Publishers
199 W. 8th Ave., Suite 3
Eugene, OR 97401

www.wipfandstock.com

ISBN 13: 978-1-62032-561-2

Cataloguing-in-Publication data:

Dobson, Melanie L.

    Health as a virtue : Thomas Aquinas and the practice of habits of health / Melanie L. Dobson.

    xiv + 146 pp. ; 23 cm. Includes bibliographical references and indexes.

    Princeton Theological Monograph Series 209

    ISBN 13: 978-1-62032-561-2

    1. Thomas, Aquinas, Saint, 1225?–1274. 2. Health—Theology. I. Title. II. Series.

B765.T54 D63 2014

Manufactured in the U.S.A.

For my parents, Robert and Lynn Dobson

Contents

Preface ix

Acknowledgments xi

PART ONE: Thomas Aquinas and Habits of Health

1. Introduction: A Story of Habits Learned   3
2. Habit and Health in Aristotelian Thought   9
3. Habit in Aquinas   17
4. Health as a Habit in Aquinas   24
5. Body, Soul, and the Healthy Life   39
6. Passionately Longing for Health   47
7. The Action of Habits of Health   54
8. What Is Health For? The Ends of Habits of Health   64

PART TWO: Habits of Health in Christian Community

9. Clergy Health Initiative   77
10. Word Made Flesh   102
11. Conclusion: Habits of Health and the Church   131

     Appendix: Interview Questions   137

     Bibliography   141
     Subject Index   147
     Names Index   155

Preface

STRUCK WITH A CHRONIC disease while in my late twenties, I decided to go back to school to read. I wanted to read everything I could about how I was to live faithfully with this disease. Books, for this bookworm, were my way to cope.

I spent over a year of my doctoral work trying to find an ethical strategy for Christian care of health. A possible answer came in my second year of reading (for which I'm profoundly grateful, otherwise I may still be in my degree program). While reading Thomas Aquinas in a Catholic Moral Theology seminar, I noticed an example repeated over and over again. In fact, in every question of Thomas's Prima Secundae questions 49–54 on Habit, references to "health" appeared. Struck by this repetition, I read these questions closely to see what, if anything, Thomas was saying about health.

This book comes out of that deep reading. Despite some inconsistencies, I believe Thomas Aquinas does indeed understand practices of health as a part of the moral life—thus contributing to how Christians might live toward a faithful life with God. How Thomas understands habit, health, and the workings of the body, soul, and heart (passions) gives support to this thesis.

I didn't want my surmise about Thomas's practices of health to only live in theory; I wanted to find embodied, communal examples of St. Thomas's insights. I did field research with United Methodist clergy participants in the Clergy Health Initiative pilot program, and with missionaries in the evangelical organization Word Made Flesh. For each I obtained an Institutional Research Board approval and used sociological methods to analyze the qualitative date from my interviews. Again, to my profound gratitude, I found that Thomas' insights actually "worked." The clergy and missionaries who engaged in habits of health, were (though not perfectly) happier, more vital human beings with improved relationships with God and greater service to others.

Preface

I offer to you, my readers, not a quick-fix diet book or exercise plan for greater physical health. To practice health as a virtue in accordance with Aquinas's thinking engages all of our being. However, flourishing with God is worth the moral effort. May you be well.

Acknowledgments

This book truly is the product of a whole community of people. First and foremost I offer gratitude to my son, Elijah. His enthusiasm for each moment, generosity of spirit, and delight in play continually remind me what flourishing looks like.

I also thank Stanley Hauerwas for patiently reading some very rough and incoherent early drafts. His steady encouragement through the long, arduous work of dissertating/bookwriting was invaluable. His critique and suggestions for improvement helped this project immensely. I'm also grateful to Amy Laura Hall for her advice and for constant support of me throughout many years of theological education. Many thanks to Allen Verhey and Ray Barfield for serving on the dissertation committee. I also offer special thanks to Duke Divinity librarian Andy Keck for steadfastly providing me with all the materials I needed for research.

I'm deeply grateful to the folks at Clergy Health Initiative for allowing me to interview their pilot participants. Many thanks go to Dr. Rae Jean Proeschold-Bell for her instructions on qualitative research and for suggestions on my interview questions. I also appreciate John James' assistance in setting up the interviews with the clergy. To the clergy whom I interviewed (who remain unnamed for confidentiality reasons) I offer my whole-hearted gratitude for your honesty and vulnerability in the interviews, and for your time. I am especially grateful for your passion and dedication in serving the challenging and oft-disregarded rural parishes.

An equal measure of thanks goes to the missionaries and staff of Word Made Flesh. Many thanks to co-director Phileena Heurtz for believing in my ability to teach yoga to evangelical Christian missionaries, and for all her support during my time at their Gathering. I thank Marcia Ghali for her logistical support in arranging for my stay with them at the Gathering and ensuring that I had all I needed. Oceans of appreciation go to the Word Made Flesh missionaries who serve Christ in destitute communities around the world. I admire your courageous lives and your commitments to sustainable, healthy lifestyles. Thank you for sharing so openly and beautifully in your interviews—and for gladly offering me

Acknowledgments

the time to interview you. Many blessings upon your work in serving the most vulnerable in our world.

To my friends in the ThD program at Duke I offer thanks for your support through the years. I'm grateful for the friendships with the people of my entering class who began this journey with me—Craig Heilmann, Warren Kinghorn, Jeff Conklin-Miller, Andrew Thompson, Denise Thorpe, Arnold Oh, and Tommy Givens. Each of you has been a gift to me. I am especially grateful for my "dissertation dialogue" group for their advice and encouragement. Many thanks to Jeff Conklin-Miller and to Rebekah Ecklund for reading/editing earlier drafts and giving suggestions, and to Heather Vacek for her steady support and stickers!

I also offer heartfelt gratitude to Daila Moreno for her dedicated love and care of my son while I worked on this book. Without her beautiful tending to Elijah, I would not have been able to finish my work. While I wrote and revised . . . and revised again, I knew my child was in gifted hands. I also thank my mom for giving so much support—and a solid week of childcare in the summer so that I could finish this project. I am so grateful!

Lastly I offer a "thanks" to the multitude of practitioners who have used their gifts to nurture health within me—from neurologists to massage therapists, from acupuncturists to physical therapists. From these dedicated people I have experienced virtuous healthcare—and have been encouraged to continue in my own practice of habits of health.

PART ONE

Thomas Aquinas and Habits of Health

1

Introduction: A Story of Habits Learned

MY LIFE, THOUGH I DIDN'T KNOW IT AT THE TIME, BROKE INTO "BEFORE" and "after."

In April 2003 as the cacti in the Sonoran desert bloomed, I sat in Dr. Schwengel's (D.O.) office in Mesa, AZ. I explained to him a searing pain in my cervical spine and my loss of control of my right leg; a couple of weeks before this visit I had been running on the desert trail near my home in the early morning and inexplicably sprained my ankle badly. Even after I stopped hobbling around on crutches my gait involved a significant limp on the right side, while my left side remained quite numb.

After explaining these symptoms Dr. Schwengel looked at the ghostly images of my recent MRI film and saw the eerie white spots floating in space at cervical spine vertebrae four and six. He lowered the film from his eyes, saying with a warm gentleness in his voice that I would need evaluation by other doctors including a neurologist, but he could work on my neck to alleviate some of the pain. When I asked what he thought of the film, he cautiously offered that the images could indicate many possible conditions, including multiple sclerosis. Multiple sclerosis. I wasn't really sure how to pronounce it, much less spell it; I didn't really know what the disease represented, except that it was a devastating chronic disease. These symptoms that I had thought were temporary and just required some medical quick fix now represented a future lifetime of serious illness. Life could no longer be the same; I had left the population of the well and had entered the communion of the chronically ill. I needed to lie down.

As my whole life whirled around me like a tornado, the good doctor led me to his examining room and had me lie down on the table for a brief respite. In midst of arid fear and uncertainty, water sprang up and started flowing down my cheeks, cutting rivulets across skin that suddenly felt withered and old, though I was only in my late twenties.

As Dr. Schwengel adjusted my back and spine with the osteopathic manipulative method, I consciously told myself, don't ask "why me?" Such a question appeared narcissistic and theologically misguided. The next, tightly holy response would be "why not me?" Yet as the doctor moved my neck one way and then the other and the pain throbbed at the base of my cervical spine, this question rang false as well. The real, most central question seemed to be "what is going to happen to me?" Questions which then followed in rapid succession included: "Would I be in this vortex of pain and debility forever? What kind of illness do I have; is it multiple sclerosis or something else? What do I need in order to endure through this new reality? What spiritual resources can I call upon? Why won't the two little creeks flowing down my cheeks stop flowing? Will I survive this? What about my family—and of my work at the church?" I don't want to become a burden to anyone... "Oh God, help me," I prayed. "God give me the strength that I need for whatever is before me."

After the treatment Dr. Schwengel helped me to sit up on the table, and for the first time in weeks the pain in my spine felt diminished. I offered gratitude to him and realized in that moment that I could both experience healing and still endure through ongoing pain simultaneously. I was just beginning to understand that healing would come for me in small steps, would involve my whole being (mind, body, soul), and would require great dedication.

As I checked out of Dr. Schwengel's office the nurse gave me a list of vitamins and supplements to support my beleaguered body. My eyes widened and my gut tightened as she pushed jar after jar of supplements to me. I had taken a Flintstone vitamin or two growing up, but this regimen required Herculean dedication. I wondered aloud if there were any gummy bear vitamins I could take instead and received only laughter and a curt "no." As I placed the bag filled with nutritional jars on my hip and limped out of the door I stepped into a life in which the nurture of whatever health I could have required incredible commitment; my habitual practices of avid running and eating a largely produce-based, organic diet were no longer enough.

After numerous trips to the neurologist with blood draws, lumbar puncture, and examinations, my condition nonetheless didn't fit into a diagnosis and thus I had no treatment protocol to follow even as my symptoms remained. While still popping incredible numbers of supplements

Introduction: A Story of Habits Learned

and with a strong determination to learn from whomever I could I began a long, ongoing journey to a wide variety of healers: physical therapists, integrative medical doctors, homeopaths, naturopaths, ophthalmologists, traditional Chinese medical doctor, acupuncturists, massage therapists, yoga teachers, feldenkrais practitioner, Rolfer, sports medicine doctor, hyperbaric chamber operator, holistic dentist, and a second neurologist. I learned to regard the search for a gifted healer as a prayer practice and to offer gratitude for what I garnered from each practitioner. The therapies or protocols that the healers gave me had to be practiced as a spiritual discipline; otherwise I wouldn't have the willpower to adhere to all the requirements. Whether the task was taking vitamins or giving myself an injection or performing some physical exercises, I had to cultivate them as habits which sustained my body so that I had the strength to continue pastoring my church and caring for others. Though I didn't receive physical healing from those habits the practice of them enabled me to persevere through pain, to maintain the health I did have, to have greater empathy for those living with serious illness, and to cultivate hope. The practice of habits that cultivated health enabled me to fully live in and through my chronic condition.

As I struggled to give spiritual grounding to the mundane tasks that I practiced to sustain my body, I longed for a theological account of tending to health. Though I knew the witness of martyrs who had sacrificed their entire lives for their faith, I also felt that the God who gives life intends for us to care for this gift. If our bodies are indeed temples, as the scriptures tell us, then those temples require good housekeeping to remain functional. I yearned for an explication of caring for my body that regarded such a practice, when kept in balance and away from narcissism, as holy. I wanted all the effort spent going to healers and practicing their regimens to be understood not as self-serving or as survival but rather as faithful.

A Story of Faith and Habit

How are we to care for our bodies and our health as a part of faithful Christian living? Such a conversation in the church is certainly fraught with difficulties, since we can hardly talk about the body without mentioning sickness and disease and we have allowed the theological vocabulary of corporeality to be replaced by modern medicine's impersonal,

PART ONE—Thomas Aquinas and Habits of Health

instrumental understanding of the body.[1] However, such lapses and the deep ambiguity in the church's history regarding embodiment exhibits the profound need for discussion. Christians remain confused about how the care of their health relates to their life of faith. We need a story that teaches us how the quotidian nurture of our beings fosters within us a greater love of God and neighbor.

Nestled within the depths of the *Summa Theologiae* Saint Thomas Aquinas offers us the outline of such a story in his questions on habit. His theology of habit offers a healthy alternative for contemporary Christians struggling to live whole lives in an era of chronic disease and a bewildering array of health/diet/exercise advice. In contrast to extremely ascetic diet and fitness programs that often result in failure, habit enables an agent to act well consistently, successfully, and with ease--without the exertion of constant moral deliberation and reasoning.[2]

As Aquinas understands them, habits are particular qualities or characteristics that accrue to a person after he or she has acted a certain way over a period of time.[3] Good habits give us the ability to act well when oriented to the performance of our proper function and created end, which leads to a virtuous life (if we practice habits that ruin our functioning and keep us from loving God, these habits result in vice. Such vicious habits cannot nurture health).[4] Through long and consistent practice habits become natural and enduring to a person—almost like his quasi-nature. Habits come to make an individual who he is; habits capture what our behavior makes of us. In the Latin *habitus*, the same word from which we derive "habitat," indicates that habits describe how we dwell in life. For Thomas good habits are virtues that offer us the ability to transform into our best selves and become more like Christ. Habit comprises not yet another diet/exercise program or solution to obesity—habits offer instead the possibility of true transformation. They direct us into deepest happiness and a life of flourishing with God. A Thomist account of habit gives Christians a theology for the cultivation of health as an element of the faithful life in the midst of a very sick world.

In order to fully explore this story of habit that Aquinas offers to us (in I-II qq 49–54), I'll first look at the classical roots of habit in

1. Shuman, *The Body of Compassion*, 6–9; McKenny, *To Relieve the Human Condition*, 21.

2. I am dependent in this definition upon Klubertanz, *Habits and Virtues*.

3. Aquinas, *Summa Theologiae* I-II 49.1.

4. Ibid., I-II 49.4, 55.3.

Introduction: A Story of Habits Learned

Aristotelian thought (chapter 2). Aristotle's understanding of habit and the cultivation of virtue, I'll argue, can encompass practices of health. Aquinas adopts key aspects of Aristotelian notions of good habit—stability, action-orientation, repetition—and adds the possibility of infused virtue and a *telos* oriented to God (chapter 3). Thus, Thomas provides a moral approach for Christians in which the cultivation of habits that sustain good health constitutes part of the virtuous life with God (chapter 4).

This life with God is a holistic one for Thomas—one that necessarily includes body and soul. Aquinas, by parsing out different kinds of habit in the body and soul (entitative versus operative) allows that the body does indeed participate in habit. This insight, coupled with Thomas's holistic anthropology, means that habits of health incorporate all of our being—body and soul. Bodies, for Aquinas, orient to God. This means our bodies, just as our souls, are for beatitude with God (chapter 5).

The interwoven nature of body and soul in habits of health includes our emotions. Thomas believes we are creatures who must feel in order to act. Over those feelings we retain moral responsibility—and ultimately those emotions yearn for the complete love we only find in God. Our yearnings for a healthier, fuller life motivate us to habits of health that ultimately enable us to land in the lap of God.

Having argued for what habits of health are and how they incorporate our whole selves (mind, body, and heart), you might want to know "how to" nurture this wonderful moral life that leads to flourishing. Obligingly, I'll show how reason and will function to help us launch a new habit of health. This action will be placed in conversation with a psychological account from J. Prochaska, J. Norcross, and C. DiClemento that offers practical, contemporary template for the action of developing healthy habits. I'll use an example of the practice of running to make the action of habit come alive (chapter 7).

The whole discussion of habits thus far leads to the end of habits of health—which for Aquinas is God. Getting to the end (both of the discussion of Aquinas and the *telos* of God) involves a deeper discussion of the journey of the virtuous life. This journey to happiness with God includes the theological and cardinal virtues. Chapter 8 explores those virtues and then leaves us at the destination of any and all habits of health—the heart of God.

In chapters 9 and 10 I'll examine two actual ministries that are implementing good habits of health as part of the life of Christian virtue. These chapters consist of an analysis of fieldwork with missionaries of

PART ONE—Thomas Aquinas and Habits of Health

Word Made Flesh and with United Methodist clergy in North Carolina who participated in the Clergy Health Initiative. Though not purposely Thomist, these two faith groups exemplify transformations wrought by the intentional practice of habits that sustain good health. This chapter demonstrates that Thomas's theology of habit provides a hermeneutic to interpret why people in these programs became happier, vibrant, and more virtuous human beings in deeper love with God.

In sum, Aquinas offers an account of health as virtue determined habitually. Thomas's understanding of habits offers a holistic approach to the tending of body and soul such that we live our best lives possible to the glory of God. In the end, unlike the ascetic practices of contemporary diet books (Christian and secular) that often lead people into despair, Aquinas's understanding of the role of virtue in health directs us into deeper joy and happiness.[5] Thomas offers that our transformation to healthier people occurs not through fad diets, weight loss programs, or specific fitness regimens, but through our life-long participation in habits oriented teleologically to love God and our neighbor. The theology of habits of health means that our quotidian care of our bodies is not only faithful, but directs us toward becoming more virtuous people who love others and God with greater joy.

---

5. Torrell, *Aquinas's Summa*, 40. Torrell offers the insight that Thomas's orientation is to the positive. Though he recognizes sin, Thomas upholds the power of God's grace. This is a marked contrast to the impulses undergirding much of the Christian "self-improvement" dieting books, which strongly emphasize sinfulness in eating. Griffiths, *Born Again Bodies*, 207.

2

Habit and Health in Aristotelian Thought

Introduction

A DISCUSSION OF HABITS OF VIRTUE, AND HEALTH AS PART OF THAT LIFE OF virtue, is best grounded in the classical theorist of virtue ethics, Aristotle. Aristotle, the son of a doctor, employed numerous healthcare analogies in his work on ethics—a long-traditioned practice among philosophers from Homer to Socrates.[1] He utilized this analogy to construct an eminently practical philosophical approach that relates to human hopes, desires and dreams, and responds to the complexity of life.[2] Aristotle felt that the good life must be attainable for any citizen through learning and effort, and that ethics must offer a person a complete existence with family, friends, and civic life.

For Aristotle, part of the good life included health. In truth, Aristotle understood "habit" and the cultivation of virtue to also encompass healthy practices. These healthy practices were supported and sustained by Aristotle's philosophy of healthcare, which allowed for a *telos* toward the divine. In order to unpack the relationship of habit, virtue, and healthcare in Aristotle, we'll first look at what the great philosopher means by habit and virtue, then connect it to a virtuous practice of health. Lastly, we'll explore how Aristotle's philosophy provides room for a healthcare that ends in contemplation of God.

---

1. Nussbaum, *Therapy of Desire*, 48–52. For example Empedocles wrote in a philosophical poem that the *logos* serves as a healer for the intellect and emotions. The *logoi* were understood by Socrates and Plato to serve as drugs for the soul. The *logos* was portrayed by Greek philosophers as the remedy for the illnesses of the soul like medical treatment remedied the illnesses of the body.

2. Aristotle, *Eudemian Ethics*, 1099b18–20.

PART ONE—Thomas Aquinas and Habits of Health

Habit and Virtue

Aristotle believes that moral virtue comes, not from a hereditary disposition or natural talent, but from practice through our nature. "So virtues arise in us neither by nature nor against nature. Rather, we are by nature able to acquire them, and we are completed through habit."[3] Humanity, in its very nature, requires habit in order to live a successful and consistent life in the midst of overwhelming options. Since habit comprises part of human nature, Aristotle thinks people must then be able muster the gumption to practice good habits and live into virtue.

He describes this practice as a quotidian activity that eventually forms us into who we are. Habit develops through repeated action and those actions indelibly form us.[4] According to Aristotle, the character of our activities shapes our own character. "A state of character results from the repetition of similar activities."[5] Such a *habitus* results from long conditioning and practice and is difficult to change.[6]

Therefore, this kind of active virtue Aristotle considered as *character* virtue. In contrast to intellectual virtues, which described states of the rational element of the soul, character virtues are states of the appetitive part of the nonrational soul. Character virtue describes our *habitus*, formed by our chosen actions.[7] As we continually repeat those actions, our virtue becomes deeply embedded and stable within us. For Aristotle, this means that by exercising virtues as active agents, we acquire them. We become just by doing just actions, courageous by doing acts of courage, and healthy from doing acts which support health; we do what is virtuous *because* it is virtuous.[8] Through the practice of good habits we become good (virtuous) and our character and work likewise.[9]

---

3. Aristotle, *Nicomachean Ethics* II, 1 (1103b).

4. Ibid., II, 1 (1103a 31–b2).

5. Ibid., II, 1 (1103a–b). "Virtues, by contrast, we acquire, just as we acquire crafts, by having first activated them. For we learn a craft by producing the same product that we must produce when we have learned it; we become builders, for instance, by building, and we become harpists by playing the harp." Aristotle discusses the importance of being apprenticed in a trade as a way of describing the training required in order to follow the virtuous habits of life.

6. Kent, "Habits and Virtues," 117.

7. Cates, *Choosing to Feel*, 6.

8. Ibid. Aristotle repeats the notion that by habit, by doing just actions one becomes just, etc. in *Nicomachean Ethics*, II, 4 (1105b); MacIntyre, *After Virtue*, 149.

9. Aristotle, *Nicomachean Ethics* 11, 6 (1106a15).

The practice of good habits also maintain the virtues once they are acquired through the "quasi-permanent quality" of the habit; "the activities of the virtues [once we have acquired them] also consist in these same actions."[10] Virtues as a habitual disposition become so deeply embedded within us that we remain stable and resist change.[11] For Aristotle, there is no way to achieve the good life as a virtuous Athenian citizen without consistently exercising the virtues through the regular practice of stable habits.[12]

The cultivation of a good life results in an end of *eudaimonia*, or the art of living well in accordance with perfect virtue.[13] For Aristotle, habits end in a *telos* of a good life as a citizen of the polis. A life of virtue ends in a life of flourishing. Aristotle provides a moral framework in which the person's very character resembles the virtuous practices that they do—practices that lead them into the art of living well (or *eudaimonia*).

Health

For Aristotle, this virtuous doing includes practices of health.[14] He often uses healthcare as a metaphor for soulcare. For example, he states that those who do not do virtuous actions are like "a sick person who listens attentively to the doctor, but acts on none of his instructions. Such a course of treatment will not improve the state of the sick person's

---

10. Aristotle, *Categories* 8 (9a3; a 9). Aristotle, *Nicomachean Ethics* II, 2 (1104b). Aristotle elaborates that "for abstaining from pleasures makes us become temperate, and once we have become temperate we are most capable of abstaining from pleasures. It is similar with bravery; habituation in disdain for frightening situations and in standing firm against them makes us become brave, and once we have become brave we shall be most capable of standing firm."

11. Cates, *Choosing to Feel*, 7.

12. MacIntyre, *After Virtue*, 149. "Within an Aristotelian framework the suggestion that there might be some means to achieve the good without the exercise of the virtues makes no sense."

13. Aristotle, *Nicomachean Ethics* (1098b 21–23).

14. Aristotle's own thought on medicine would have undoubtedly been shaped by his father, a physician. He would have learned medicine from the Hippocratic corpus, in which the body was understood to be constituted by four elements, or humors: black bile, yellow bile, and phlegm, which needed to be in proportion and balance to one another in order for a person to be healthy. The four humors were then adapted to the seasons, winds, and elements (earth, air, fire, water) through the artful practice of a physician in order to describe and accommodate disease. Porter, *Flesh in the Age of Reason*, 49. See also University of Virginia Health System, "Hippocrates."

PART ONE—Thomas Aquinas and Habits of Health

body; nor will the many improve the state of their souls by this attitude to philosophy."[15] For Aristotle, the action of caring for one's health parallels the action of caring for one's soul.

An Aristotelian understanding of health orients to the mean—neither excess or deficiency—just like any other practice in the virtuous life.[16] The philosopher argues that the mean is determined by each person's nature and practices—so that what would be sufficient food for a gymnast might be excessive for a non-athlete.[17] In the *Nicomachean Ethics* he connects healthcare practices in the mean to virtue: "For both excessive and deficient exercise ruin bodily strength, and similarly, too much or too little eating or drinking ruins health, whereas the proportionate amount produces, increases, or preserves it. The same is true, then, of temperance, bravery, and the other virtues."[18] Through the exercise of habits that are balanced, we subsequently live healthier lives. Thus, Aristotle offers the example of walking; through a balanced (neither too extreme or too lax) practice of walking, we become healthy walkers . . . and more virtuous people in the process.[19]

Therefore, Aristotle combines the character-building practice of habit with balanced (in the mean) actions like walking and exercise to provide a moral basis for the care of health. This healthcare empowers people to be active agents both morally and physically in tending to their wellbeing—a tending that actually ends in more virtuous, happy lives. Aristotle's epistemology grounded in habits supports a life of virtue that includes practices toward greater health.

The Ends of Healthcare—Health as a Product versus Health as Practice of Virtue

Aristotle's understanding of practices of health as a part of the virtuous life participates in his philosophical understanding of healthcare. The

---

15. Aristotle, *Nicomachean Ethics* II 4 (1105a), 22.

16. Ibid., (1106b 20). The mean consists of acting "at the right times, with reference to the right objects, towards the right people, with the right motive, and in the right way."

17. Ibid., II 6 (1106b 35). Here he offers the example that a gymnast athlete will require more food than a person who doesn't train as intensely.

18. Ibid., II, 2 (1104a). "Temperance and bravery, then, are ruined by excess and deficiency, but preserved by the mean."

19. Ibid., V, 1 (1129a).

philosopher primarily understood healthcare as comprised of ancillary science. However, as will be argued here, ultimate science, since it leads to a life of flourishing, must also be considered part of healthcare in Aristotelian thought. Below we'll explore his understanding of ancillary science, which utilizes *techne* and in which health can only be considered a product of a craft. On the other hand, ultimate science, which includes the pursuit of virtue, allows for healthcare to be virtuous as a habitual practice. The distinction in these two sciences allows for a practice of healthcare that leads to an end (*telos*) of a virtuous life.

Ancillary Science and Techne

Aristotle understood science as being of two categories, the first being "ancillary science"; this science deals with the utilitarian and productive aspects of the cosmos. Within ancillary science humans, utilizing reason, can understand and participate in the particular and normative order of the cosmos.[20] Aristotle understood reason's purpose as providing humanity with greater synchronization and awareness of the cosmic order. People deploy reason, particularly scientific reason, through the senses, feelings, and intuition in order to better understand the world around them. Within ancillary science artisans use their reason through their senses in order to craft and produce products.

Aristotle has a term for the making of a product; he called this skill of crafting *techne*. He understood doctors as producing (*poieseis*) health through the practice of their *techne* (craft).[21] As a *techne*, medicinal artisans understood health as a standard for bodily excellence; the task of the doctor was to determine the nature and degree of health with reference to each person. This *techne* required not only anatomical knowledge but also insight into the capacity of a particular patient. Excellence for any patient involved a harmony of body/mind/spirit, tempered with the clear understanding that human beings were mortals destined to suffer disease and die.[22]

---

20. The order in which the moon travels around the earth, the order in the manner in which plants grow, and the patterns in the ways humans mature all demonstrate the normative order of the cosmos.

21. Knight, *Aristotelian Philosophy*, 17, 26; Aristotle, *Nicomachean Ethics* VI 4.4, 88.

22. McKenny, *To Relieve the Human Condition*, 16.

For Aristotle the production (*poiesis*) of health by the *techne* of doctors reproduces pre-existing forms—it constitutes a good to be produced by a process.[23] The doctor is simply a means to health; he or she represents the source/agent for change for the sake of the individual patient and for the universal form of human health.[24] Medical practitioners don't deliberate or contemplate in their production of cures; instead he or she lays down the end of health and examines ways and means to achieve it.[25]

However, for Aristotle the production of the external good of health through a *techne*, as is the work of medicine, allows only for an instrumental goodness. The practices of the art of medicine produce one end—bodily health.[26] The external good of health is indeed necessary for a good life, but isn't entirely sufficient. Therefore, according to Aristotle, those doctors who live a life of labor producing external goods of health are unable to cultivate the internal goods of virtue (*arête*) and live full lives of excellence.[27] Their patients, who receive the good of bodily health from their doctor's practice of *techne*, have received a worthy product (health)—but aren't necessarily any further along on the journey of virtue. This means that for Aristotelian philosophy based only in ancillary science, practitioners of medicine and their patients are unable to be virtuous; his understanding of *techne* as production keeps them from such pursuits. Health understood only as a product, then can't be virtuous.

Ultimate Science and Theoria

However, Aristotle provides a pathway for the cultivation of virtue (*arête*) in the healthcare of the body through his understanding of "ultimate science." Ultimate science has a primary concern for wonderment at the cosmos (rather than investigation) and contemplation of the Divine. This most honorable and supreme science deals with divine objects and first

---

23. Knight, *Aristotelian Philosophy*, 10. This process could be taking a walk or getting some sort of treatment.

24. Ibid., 11. The doctor is the external producer of health, but his practice is not for his own sake as a doctor but for the universal form of a healthy human being. In the same way when a builder builds the work produced is for the sake of bringing into existence the form of the house—it isn't for the builder per se.

25. Aristotle, *Nicomachean Ethics* III 3.11, 35.

26. Nussbaum, *The Therapy of Desire*, 74–75.

27. Knight, *Aristotelian Philosophy*, 26. Aristotle, *Nicomachean Ethics* 1, 6.10–11. Aristotle offers that external goods obtain their goodness from internal goods, deriving his argument from Plato.

Habit and Health in Aristotelian Thought

principals from God and exists in the realm of the supernatural; it is also known as theology or Wisdom.

Ultimate science encourages the focus upon God while letting go of scientific rationality—a focus that Aristotle calls *theoria*. Aristotle understands that human beings are to imitate God, the prime mover and complete end (*telos*). Beings imitate God by engaging in *energeia* (activity characteristic of a being's kind) in order to actualize their good (*telos*) by contemplating the divine.[28] As the most self-sufficient and complete activity available to us *theoria* leads us into the best life possible—a life of leisured contemplation of that which is unchanging and which leads to *eudaimonia*.[29] *Eudaimonia*, or the activity of living well and doing well, equates to a life of full flourishing.[30] Such happiness comes because the activity of *theoria* is completely unproductive—if it were a means to some further end it could not be our *telos*.

The practice of habits, which when activated lead to virtue (*arête*) certainly comprise *energeia*, since habits form us into who we are—and the definition of *energia* is activity characteristic of a being's kind. Since health can be considered a habit that leads to virtue, the practice of health as a habit then can help humans to actualize their good, or *telos*. Therefore, habits of health as virtuous practice oriented to our *telos* of contemplation of God can help to direct us to *eudaimonia*. Healthcare as a virtuous practice can participate in ultimate science and lead humans to flourishing.

Some discrepancy does exist in Aristotle on the practice of health versus the production of health as a part of the virtuous life. Aristotle contradicts himself on the possibility of virtue in healthcare with inconsistent distinctions between *poiesis* (production) and *praxis* (action).[31] Nonetheless, even if a doctor's *techne* results in productivity, that skill could still be controlled and directed by a *praxis* of contemplation

28. Knight, *Aristotelian Philosophy*, 7. "It is in contemplating the divine that humans come the closest of which they are capable to participating in divinity."

29. Aristotle, *Nicomachean Ethics* X 6–8.

30. Ibid., II (1102a5). See also Cates, *Choosing to Feel*, 5-6.

31. For example in book 6 of *Nicomachean Ethics* Aristotle states that doctoring doesn't direct health but is for the sake of bringing health into being, distinguishing practice from theory. *NE* 1145a6–8. In *NE* VII (*NE* 1147a28–30) he offers in an example concerned with nutrition and the production of health a contrast between productive activity and theoretical reasoning. The interpretation of Aristotle's distinctions between *praxis* and *poiesis* has a long and storied history, which is much longer and more complex than can be documented here.

PART ONE—Thomas Aquinas and Habits of Health

independent from the product (health) produced by the craft.[32] If a medical practitioner can deliberate upon the ultimate *telos* rather than just engage in technical productivity, he or she could cultivate *arête*. Thus, patients and healthcare practitioners could both participate in ultimate science and nurture lives of flourishing by engaging in health as a practice, rather than just a product.

Conclusion

According to Aristotle, the cultivation of good habits constitutes a necessary step toward the possibility of a life of *arête* and of flourishing. In his philosophical framework care of one's health can be included as a practice that shapes one's character, and directs a person to a more virtuous life. The care of the body, like the care of the soul, leads to *eudiamonia*. Health as a virtuous practice contributes to one's ability to contemplate God (*theoria*), and live the best life possible.

Aristotle's philosophy of habit will then provide the basis for Thomas Aquinas's adaptation to a Christian audience. For Thomas the Aristotelian cultivation of virtue through habit ultimately directs practitioners to the God revealed in Jesus Christ. The Christian understanding of Aristotelian habit affirms the importance of agency, while at the same time pointing beyond the individual practitioner to a life of flourishing with God and others in a loving community. Aquinas would take Aristotle's understanding of habit as including health and develop it further for the Christian life—a development explored in the next chapters.

---

32. Knight, *Aristotelian Philosophy*, 25. Knight cites C. D. C. Reeve as offering this theory.

3

Habit in Aquinas

Introduction

THOMAS AQUINAS, A DOMINICAN PREACHER AND CONSUMMATE THEOlogian from the twelfth century, takes up Aristotle's writings on habit in questions 49-54 in the Prima Secundae of his *Summa Theologiae*. Aquinas will expand and develop these notions of habit from Aristotle, but will also add his own Christian interpretation.

A Thomistic understanding of habits includes them as a necessary part of the virtuous life (as did Aristotle). Aquinas agrees with Aristotle that human beings by their nature have the agency (gumption) to practice habit. Thomas offers that the pluripotent nature of human life makes it necessary for habit to exist in order for people to direct action toward a good end. Habit enables humans to act well, consistently and successfully—without having to expend considerable deliberative effort and reasoning for each act amidst an exorbitant array of options.[1] Human will isn't taxed as much in habit as it is with deliberative action, so human nature really needs habit in order to function well.[2]

Below we'll consider Aquinas's use and adaptation of Aristotle on habit. Aquinas corroborates Aristotle on habits as having a lastingness

1. Aquinas, *Summa Theologiae*, I-II 49.3 and I-II 49.4. see also I-IIae 55.1 All references to the *Summa Theologiae* come from this translation (Cambridge University Press) unless otherwise noted. Dunnington, "Addiction and Action," 40.

2. Dunnington, "Addiction and Action," 44. see also Putnam, "The Moral Life of a Pragmatist," as quoted in Shuman, *Body of Compassion*, 119. "A well-established routine becomes a habit, and a firm habit will, in novel circumstances, establish a routine. What routines and habits do for us is this: they obviate the necessity to decide at every moment what to do next; they provide an easy explanation for a host of actions." See also Klubertanz, *Habits and Virtues*.

that shapes our character, as formed by action, as repetitive, as able to be increased/decreased/corrupted, and as capable of disposing us to virtue. Aquinas also adds that habits may be infused by grace and have a *telos* oriented to God. This close reading of Aquinas's understanding of habit provides the ethical foundation to be developed throughout the rest of the book.[3]

Habit as a Lasting Quality

For Aristotle, habits retain a "quasi-permanent quality"; this stability allows for us as human beings to resist change and develop character.[4] Likewise, Aquinas refers to habits as "quasi-permanent" and not easily lost.[5] Aquinas differentiates habit's quality of permanence from a "state," which is easily lost. He uses the example of a transitory illness as a state, and knowledge and virtue as habits.[6] These habits are attributes of a person that concern their nature. Habits, in effect, help to make us who we are; they indicate our character—because they are lasting and stable within us.

Habit as Formed by Action

The gumption, or agency, in habit comes through action for Aquinas. He quotes Augustine that "a habit is something which permits action at need."[7] He follows by stating that "intrinsically, every habit is in some way connected with action."[8] Habits don't constitute the activity itself; it is instead the potential with respect to activity.[9] For Aquinas, like Aristotle,

---

3. The ordering of these seven descriptors of habit derive from the way Aquinas develops his understanding of habit in his Treatise on Habit. I'm simply following his development of habit.

4. Cates, *Choosing to Feel*, 7.

5. Aquinas, *ST* I-II 49.3.

6. Aquinas is working with Aristotle's *Categories* here, and places habit in the first type of quality. Aristotle's classification has problems, as some qualities can fit in one or more categories. There are different possibilities given by Aristotle for the difference between a state and a habit. Aquinas, *ST* 22.115–16.

7. Augustine, *De Bono Coniugali*, as quoted in Aquinas, *ST* I-II 49.3 sed contra.

8. Aquinas, *ST* I-II 49. 3.

9. Ibid. Aquinas is utilizing Aristotle, *On the Soul* II, 1 (412a 22) here. Oesterle gives the example in which science is a habit. The first act (habit) is the possession of knowledge, the second act would be the exercise of the knowledge or science. Aquinas,

humans have the capacity to initiate habit's potential to live more virtuous lives.[10]

Habit Bears Repeating

Aquinas affirms Aristotle's insight that habit is formed by repetitive action.[11] "After repeated action, a certain quality is produced in the passive potentiality which is acted upon, and it is this quality which is called a habit."[12] In effect then, "habits capture what our behavior makes of us."[13] For Aquinas, like Aristotle, our actions and behavior mark us with certain traits over time so that we become what we most consistently and repeatedly do. If we do healthy acts (which Aquinas uses copiously as an example), then we become healthy.

Habit Can Be Increased, Decreased, Corrupted

However, even though habits provide stable qualities, they themselves can increase, decrease, or be corrupted, according to Aristotle, and

---

Treastise on the Virtues, 8 n. 50.

10. Aquinas, *ST* I-II 50.3 Aquinas clarifies here that habit as part of human nature is not equivalent with natural instinct or powers. Sense powers operating according to natural instinct cannot possess habit because they are oriented only to one thing. Instinct functions apart from reason within the nutritive part of the soul. Without any potential for different actions, instinct remains incapable of habit.

11. Aristotle, *Nicomachean Ethics* II, 1 (1103a 31–b2) as cited by Aquinas, I-II 51. 2. "Aristotle teaches that virtuous and vicious habits are caused by action." However, Aquinas is careful to say here that habits do not form from acts in an agent in which there is only an active principle (for example in fire there is only the active principle of heating). He is careful to indicate that habits require an agent in which there is an active and passive principle for action—as is the case for human beings.

12. Aquinas, *ST* I-II 51.2 Aquinas goes on here to say that "in the same way the habits which constitute the moral virtues are produced in the appetitive faculties when these are acted upon by reason; and the habits which constitute scientific knowledge are produced in the mind in so far as it is acted up by the primary propositions." Habits of moral virtue will be the ones we are most concerned with in regards to the body, for habits of the intellect do not include the body for Aquinas. Since habits of moral virtue are caused in appetitive powers as moved by reason and reason is unable to dominate an appetitive power in just one act, Aquinas teaches that the action must be repeated many times in order for it to be impressed firmly upon the memory. Aquinas, I-IIae 51.2–3.

13. Wadell, *The Primacy of Love*, 113.

subsequently Aquinas.[14] Aquinas offers that they can be increased, not by more substance, but by the habits themselves.[15] Secondly, habits can be increased by the subject's participation in the habit.[16] Through a subject's more intense participation in a particular habit, that habit produces a more perfect participation in an existing form.[17] Habits increase only when the intensity of the act equals or exceeds the intensity of the existing habit; with such repeated acts of higher/equal to intensity the habit grows.[18] Like Aristotle, Aquinas believes that habits can also be corrupted; they are susceptible to diminishment through the way in which the subject participates and through a cessation of the act.[19] If a person participates with less intensity than that with which the habit began, the habit diminishes. He writes, "the habit grows stronger when a lot of actions have been performed. If, on the other hand, the strength of the action is proportionately less than the strength of the corresponding habit, then the action does not help the habit to grow stronger but prepares its decay."[20] The actual action resulting from the habit must equal the potentiality of the habit if the habit is to be maintained. The interior quality of the habit must equal the exterior act; without an equal interior "intensity" of intent and desire the habit just conditions but doesn't habituate and is eventually lessened in intensity.[21]

Habit, in other words, requires continual, balanced action in order to be maintained, or it is lost or diminished. If a person begins a habit

---

14. Aquinas, *ST* I-II 52.1. For Aristotle and Aquinas the species of a thing must remain fixed and constant–habit doesn't change the species of the participant. Aristotle, *Metaphysics*, 3 (1044a 10). Since habits are ordered to something (to good in the case of virtue), they don't maintain substance in and of themselves.

15. Aquinas *ST* I-II 52.1. "First, in themselves, as we speak of greater and lesser health, and greater and lesser knowledge."

16. Ibid.

17. Ibid., I-II 52.2 The habit doesn't increase by an addition to the form (actual thing). Such additions of form to form would change the species of a thing—like going from the color tan to white.

18. Ibid., I-II 52.3. This is to say that not every act increases a habit if it is of lesser intensity.

19. Ibid., I-II 53.2 and I-II 53.3.

20. Ibid., I-II 52. 3.

21. Ibid., I-II 52.3. Also Dunnington, "Addiction and Action," 56. Though it takes many acts, for example, to make one just, a person can lapse into becoming an unjust person through lack of attention to oppressive circumstances, or through resuming behaviors that commit injustice.

with great enthusiasm, and maintains and even increases her commitment to the habit, the habit grows to become a part of her character/life. If, however, she begins the habit, but enthusiasm wanes, and she drops off in her practice, then the habit fades away. In sum, Aquinas affirms what Aristotle established on people's ability to change or lose their habits.

Habit Disposes Us to Virtue

Again corroborating Aristotle, Aquinas argues that those habits that dispose us to the good are called virtues and the human production of good habits leads to virtue.[22] "For this reason the virtue of anything has to be judged in reference to a good. Human virtue, therefore, which is an operative habit, is a good habit and productive of the good."[23]

Aquinas also expands Aristotle's point that "the exercise of good habits equals virtue" by requiring integrity all the way through the action. Not only must the external act be good, but for Aquinas even the interior commitment behind the act must be good. In other words, a person isn't virtuous just because she is adept and has abilities for good work—she must also use her aptitude and abilities rightly toward the good.[24] A virtuous person not only does good acts well that are oriented to the good, but her goodness abides in her person.[25] In colloquial language, she is good "inside and out."

Habits as Infused by Grace

In the subsequent two aspects of habit, though, Thomas deviates from Aristotle. He articulates an understanding of habit for Christian practitioners. By so doing he offers a tactical practice that empowers Christians to be faithful to Christ in their cultivation of virtue. To begin with,

22. Aquinas, *ST* I-II 49.3, 55.1. Virtue indicates a perfection of a power, and the height of any power must be good, since evil indicates a defect. Aquinas, *ST*, I-II 55.3 translated W. D. Hughes, volume 23 (Ia2ae 55–67). Aquinas quotes Dionysius here to state that every evil indicates a weakness in Dionysius, *The Divine Names* IV, 32.

23. Aquinas, *ST* I-II 55.3 Aquinas quotes Aristotle in the sed contra to this same meaning: "virtue is what makes its possessor good and his work good likewise." Aristotle, *Nicomachean Ethics* II, 6. 1106a15.

24. Therefore a brilliant scientist could use his adept skills to create something harmful rather than helpful to humanity. Just because a person is good at something doesn't make that person good.

25. Mattison, *Introducing Moral Theology*, 63.

PART ONE—Thomas Aquinas and Habits of Health

Thomas understands that some habits are infused by grace into human beings in order that they may be disposed to the proper, perfect end—the end being "final and perfect happiness for human beings."[26] Habits that dispose to such a superhuman end must exceed the power of human nature, since habits must be proportionate to what a person is disposed to by them. Therefore, superhuman habits require the infusion of grace by God. These infused habits, such as the theological virtues of faith, hope, and charity, are given to us as gifts that draw us nearer to God. Thomas clarifies the gift of infused grace by stating that "acts produced by an infused habit do not cause a habit, but strengthen the habit already existing"[27] By strengthening our ability to practice habits of love and goodness, God enables us to be people of habit who live our life toward our Creator in the world.[28]

Habits With an End in God

Secondly, Aquinas adapts Aristotle's teleological understanding of habit by understanding God as the end of our virtuous life.[29] Virtuous habits order us to the joy and happiness of friendship with God. This "happiness is gradually, sometimes painstakingly, attained. It is the work of a virtuous lifetime."[30] Habits dispose us to valuable ends—to friendship with the One who created us.[31] The strategy of Thomist ethics on habit is the

---

26. Aquinas, *ST* I-II 51.4. Thomas has also stated this end in I-II 5.5. We should clarify that Aristotle didn't conceive of theological virtues or their infusion into human beings; Thomas gets this idea from Peter Lombard's *Sentences*. Kent, "Habits and Virtues," 119.

27. Aquinas, *ST* I-II 51.4. However, Thomas also argues that God can "produce the effects of secondary causes without the secondary causes themselves." Aquinas also stated this idea in I 105. 6. He offers the example of God giving the apostles a gift of scriptural and language knowledge, which they didn't acquire through their own effort. In granting such gifts of habits that could have been caused by people's own natural powers and efforts, God doesn't go against nature. God grants gifts of habit to some (and not to others) out of God's own inscrutable wisdom. God's infusion of habit, whether for the virtues of faith, hope, and charity or by granting habits to those who didn't cultivate them through natural powers, indicates God's participation in and support of the human life of virtue.

28. Wadell, *Primacy of Love*, 115.

29. Torrell, *Aquinas's Summa*, 32.

30. Wadell, *Primacy of Love*, 59.

31. Shuman, *Body of Compassion*, 119.

Habit in Aquinas

total transformation of ourselves into people who can truly call God's kingdom our home. Habits change us into our most blessed possibility.[32]

In summation Aquinas adopts the primary aspects of Aristotelian notions of good habit—stable, consisting of action, repetitive, stable, virtuous—and includes infused virtues and a *telos* oriented to God to create a Christian practice of *habitus*. Thomas's moral strategy unites us with the God whose love has made us and will not let us go; it teaches us how to live so that we can return to God.[33] Aquinas offers an ethical pathway for Christians to become more faithful to God. Thomistic habits offer us possibilities for change and growth, giving us hope for improvement to become more Christ-like in our actions and being.[34]

With a full understanding of what Thomas means by Aristotelian notions of habit, we'll next explore health as a kind of habit that deepens our life of virtue. The practice of Thomistic habits of health enables us to draw closer to our God who is the source of all things good---—a journey that promotes healing even for the chronically ill.

---

32. Wadell, *Primacy of Love*, 113. Habit can also orient us to proximate ends. These ends are good, but don't constitute the supernatural good of beatitude with God. A good such as health would fall into this category. Thus for Aquinas there exist *teloi* within the larger *telos* of *eudaimonia* with God.

33. Wadell, *Primacy of Love*, 136.

34. Aquinas, *ST* I-II, 52. 1–2.

4

Health as a Habit in Aquinas

AQUINAS NOT ONLY DEVELOPS AND EXPANDS ARISTOTELIAN NOTIONS OF habit, he also notes Aristotle's references to health and utilizes them in his own examples of the moral life. Aquinas mentions health no less than fifteen times in his volume on habits (1a2ae 49-54). Every single question in the *Treatise on Habit* references health.[1] Like Aristotle, for Thomas it appears that a consideration of habits of virtue naturally includes a discussion of health. Aquinas states that the "virtue of anything must be expressed in terms of the good. Hence human virtue, which is an operative habit, is a good habit and productive of good works."[2] If good habits orient to virtues, and health certainly represents a good, then health must be worthy of consideration and practice. The cultivation of health embodies a moral good oriented to the kind of life God wants for us. In arguing that health constitutes a habit for Aquinas, we'll examine what Thomas means—and doesn't mean by "health." Then I'll develop chapter 2 and 3's definitions of habit in relationship to practices of health, using a case study of the exercise of running. For Thomas, the practice of health represents a vital part of the virtuous life lived to an end in God's love.

What Health Means for Aquinas

Aquinas consistently uses the Latin word *sanus/sanitatis* for health, which translated means "to be sound, healthy, sensible, and sane"—holding within the word itself ideas of both moral and physical health. Thomas

---

1. Aquinas mentions specifically mentions health in *ST* I-II 49.1-4, I-II 50.1, 3, I-II 51.1, 3-4, I-II 52.1, 2, I-II 53.1, I-II 54.1.

2. Aquinas, *Treatise on the Virtues*, I-II 55.3.

upholds Aristotle's use of health to exemplify the moral life and physical practices as orienting to the mean. Yet (as is typical for Aquinas) he nuances his understanding of health so that health's definition includes both "health as a status", and "health as an entitative habit." This nuanced and intelligent perspective on health provides for a Christian practice that acknowledges we can get sick, but won't leave us in a morass of enervating self-pity about it.

Health as a Status

Aquinas understands health as a quality that is well disposed in nature and orientation but is also easily lost.[3] In this definition, health (and sickness) by its nature has variable causes (and losses) and is properly termed a disposition, not a habit.[4] Aquinas believes that health as a status can be nourished both by exterior principles such as medicine, and/or from divine intervention; God can produce health without a natural cause in order to manifest His power.[5] Whether by nature or divine intervention, though, health can be easily changed, altered, or lost in humans. Such an orientation toward constant change means that "health as a status" cannot be a habit, since habit (as discussed above) retains a quasi-permanent status and is resistant to change.

Thomas also allows for there being variations among people's health status according to their different constitutions.[6] Though Thomas wouldn't have known concepts of heredity, he does note that some health is from "nature," meaning that someone can be genetically predisposed toward sicknesses or can have an immune system (nature) that aids one in recovering health.[7] Like Aristotle, Thomas understood "nature" as comprised of the Hippocratic humors, which need to be in correct human proportion and balance for there to be a disposition of health.[8] There

---

3. Aquinas, *ST* I-II 49.1–2.

4. Ibid., I-II 49.2.

5. Ibid., I-II 51.1, 4.

6. Ibid., I-II 51.1. "It is natural to Socrates or Plato to be sickly or healthy, according to their respective physical constitutions."

7. Ibid.

8. Aquinas, *ST* I-II 54.1; Porter, *Flesh in the Age of Reason*, 49. In this article Aquinas considers the humors in the body, and acknowledges that the balance of those humors leads to health—in the much same way as Aristotle did. Aquinas would have had Galen's anatomical canon added to the Hippocratic corpus; this medicine

can also be fluctuations in health so that it is more or less at different times in a person's life, while that person could still be said to be healthy overall.[9] In other words, for Aquinas brief illnesses don't profoundly affect one's health status. In sum, people's health according to constitution, heredity, immune system function, and temporary fluctuations can only be qualified as a status. "Health as a status" for Aquinas does not possess moral capacities.

Aquinas utilizes his understanding of the vegetative soul to affirm the absence of moral virtue in "health as a status." "The faculties of the nutrient part (of the soul) are not naturally capable of obeying the command of reason, and therefore there are no habits in them."[10] So just as habit cannot be in the body's functions (nutritive, etc) it cannot be in the health of that body.[11]

However, Thomas doesn't completely view our health as a given status. He also supports our responsibility in the care and nurture of our health; health is not just a matter of given genetic constitution. This second understanding of health does retain the moral capacities of habit, and it is to this aspect of health that we now turn.

Health as a Habit

Thomas states clearly in I-II 49 that "health is a habit," quoting Aristotle from the *Metaphysics*.[12] By this Aquinas means that health is in the first

---

would have been practiced in medieval Europe as *physic*. Also in this article Thomas offers that "if the humours are in a state which accords with human nature we have the habit or disposition of health." Does Thomas mean here that the humours, or status of the body, can be habituated—or does he mean more that the humours are a changeable, non-habitual disposition? Since at the end of the paragraph he also interchanges the terms "habit" and "disposition," I can't say for certain. However, based upon his definition of disposition as more changeable than habit, it seems most likely that the humours for Thomas comprise a status of the human that changes frequently, but can contribute to a habit of strength or weakness in the body.

9. Aquinas, *ST* I-II 52. 1.

10. Ibid., I-II 50.3.

11. Later in this chapter under the discussion of health and passions I will offer that anatomical science unavailable to Aquinas demonstrates that health of our organs/bodily functions impacts reason and thus habit—offering a correction to Aquinas's understanding of the vegetative soul.

12. Aristotle, *Metaphysics* as cited in Aquinas, *ST* I-II 49.1 and 49.4. When Aquinas states in I-II 50.1 that health is not a habit absolutely, but "like a habit" he is referring to the changeable nature of health as a status. By differentiating between health as a status

species of quality that is difficult to change—an integral part of habit's definition.[13] Health resides in the person as a habit, ordering his or her nature. A person *is* healthy according to how their condition compares to what a healthy human is determined to be (health as a status), but a person can cultivate a greater or lesser degree of health according to how they participate in their own health.[14] Health can increase or decrease by the habits that a person cultivates regarding their wellbeing.

Therefore health constitutes not just a status for Aquinas, but a moral activity in which every person participates. Health's attribute as a habit means that health, or the lack thereof, doesn't just happen to us. For Thomas we retain a Christian responsibility, regardless of our current health status, heredity, or diseased/disabled condition, to practice the care of our health.[15] Health as a habit means that how we treat our beings matters; we are not disembodied rational minds, but we are enfleshed creatures whose flesh deserves and demands virtuous attention. Health as a habit means we join with God in a journey toward the greatest wholeness and wellbeing we can experience in this life on earth.

By acknowledging health as a status Aquinas can sympathize with all those who struggle with disease etiologies outside of their control or who were born with disabilities. Yet at the same time the Thomist understanding of health as a habit exhorts these people to engage in practices that nudge them toward the most vibrant life they can have. Thomas complexifies the meaning of "health" so that it is both passive and active. Aquinas thus requires Christians to participate in their own healthcare as a part of faithful life oriented to God.

---

and health as a habit, I'm able to clarify what seems like a contradiction in Aquinas. In a subsequent section below I'll explore in more depth how health is a habit—here I'm just trying to support that health has a moral aspect to it.

13. Aquinas, *ST* I-II 50.1 Aquinas clarifies that Aristotle also places health as habit in the first species of quality (Aristotle *Physics* VII, 3 [246b 4]), in contradiction to Simplicius's argument.

14. "Health itself admits of more and less: there is not the same proportion of humours in all, nor always the same in each, but up to a point health may grow less and still be health." Aristotle, *Nicomachean Ethics*, 10, 3 (1173a24–6) as quoted in Aquinas, *ST* I-II 52.1. Clearly, Aquinas's conceptions of what health is are heavily influenced by Aristotle.

15. This perspective also affirms Barth's insistence that we are to cultivate whatever health we may have; otherwise we capitulate to the forces of death.

PART ONE—Thomas Aquinas and Habits of Health

What Health Does Not Mean for Aquinas

However, Thomas resists any vestiges of Pelagianism. He doesn't think that through our own efforts we can save ourselves from sickness and death (unlike many bestselling health self-help books). Also, unlike the bastions of modern industrial medicine that expend billions of dollars striving toward health, Thomas recognizes that health isn't the greatest good in life. Those medical complexes stand as contemporary temples to the worship of health; Aquinas's understanding of health definitively resists idolatry. As a way of further clarifying Aquinas's articulation of health, we'll argue for what a Thomistic vision of health is *not*—namely salvation, the *summum bonum*, an idol, and the definition from the World Health Organization.

Health Is Not Salvation

Aquinas states clearly that "neither man, nor any other creature, can attain ultimate happiness by his own natural powers";[16] "one needs a strength from grace that is added to natural strength for one reason, namely in order to do and wish supernatural good (ultimate happiness)."[17] Therefore for Thomas, even with our best habits of health, the perfect happiness and salvation of the afterlife comes only by grace.[18] Health cannot be conflated with salvation in Thomas.

Besides salvation being absolutely dependent upon grace, health differs from salvation in a couple more ways. Health requires personal responsibility, dedication and commitment, but such works don't require faith. Pagans can also dedicate themselves to the care of their health. Salvation, on the other hand, doesn't make sense unless one has been moved by grace to faith in Christ. "Health and salvation are also distinguished by the fact that complete health always includes physical well-being whereas salvation does not depend upon one's bodily condition. . . the Christian scriptures do not assume that vital faith in God is accompanied by physical and mental wellbeing . . ."[19] Therese of Liseaux, for example, suffered poor bodily health but was a saint who certainly rests in the bosom of God. We do not have to be perfectly healthy in order to be saved into

---

16. Aquinas, *ST* I-II 5.5.
17. Ibid., I-II 109.2 in Bauerschmidt, *Holy Teaching*, 125.
18. Kent, "Habits and Virtues," 124.
19. Evans, *Redeeming Marketplace Medicine*, 75.

Health as a Habit in Aquinas

God's perfection. For Thomas, even with our best habits of health, the perfect health, happiness and salvation of the afterlife is attainable only by grace.[20]

Health Is Not the Summum Bonum

Aquinas's understanding of virtue ethics places limits on what health can be for humans. Clearly, a Thomist understanding of ends places the greatest good squarely in the lap of God; our highest good is beautiful friendship with the Creator who made us. Although health is a good, it isn't the greatest good, or *summum bonum*. Our health and the means to it enable us to better serve God's glory, but health isn't glorious in and of itself.[21] Physical, emotional, and social health is an important good, but not the ultimate good.[22] As Thomas says, "the end is the measure of things ordered to the end", which means that health is a legitimate human end, but most be ordered properly to the ultimate end, which is human flourishing, or beatitude in God.[23]

Health Is Not an Idol

Thomas's recognition that health, while a good isn't a god, keeps Christians from worshipping health. In America health promoting habits often aren't just for well-being's sake but are also seen as a means for personal and social redemption; "wellness becomes a mechanism for the middle class... to demonstrate virtuousness while still focusing on themselves."[24] People expend astronomical sums of money and amounts of time to feel better and look good as a way of demonstrating their own worth and value. Thomas counters such Pelagianism by utilizing Aristotle's teaching on the mean—habits of health when done to the right degree lead one to God; habits when done too much or too little lead one to narcissism.

---

20. Kent, "Habits and Virtues," 124.
21. Verhey, *Reading the Bible*.
22. Shuman, *Body of Compassion*, 83.
23. Aquinas, *Treatise on Happiness*, 3. The contemporary health culture (from Weight Watchers to Gold's Gym) and many Christian-based weight loss programs lose sight of proper ends, confusing weight loss or fitness with happiness.
24. Conrad, "Wellness as Virtue," 388, 398.

PART ONE—Thomas Aquinas and Habits of Health

Health Is Not the WHO

The World Health Organization (WHO), founded in 1948, defines health as " a state of complete physical, mental, and social well-being and not merely the absence of disease or infirmity"[25] appears to be holistic and consistent with Thomistic thought. However, the WHO definition of health assumes, along with modern medicine, that we can trace illness to one germ or one gene gone wrong and then instrumentally find ways of ridding ourselves of any lingering finitude or illness.[26] Even though the WHO's definition seemingly promotes health over disease, it's still indelibly connected with a disease-care system that doesn't know how to cultivate health.

The WHO and its definition also assume the human body can be conformed to the aims of science, often without consulting the patient. "Modernity (and its medicine) purports to know with some certainty what health is, based upon scientific knowledge of the body."[27] The legacy of Enlightenment continues to haunt this WHO definition with an underlying assumption of the body as machine or product.[28] Even if scientific medicine manipulates the bodily "project" toward the good of health, it still objectifies the patient. The WHO definition doesn't convey any sense of patient agency or of their ability to cultivate their own habits of health—thus it lacks any moral foundation.

Lastly, the WHO definition lacks any larger *telos*. God and flourishing are largely exempt from this definition, except in some vague reference to the "spiritual." Such a definition would be unrecognizable as "health" for Aquinas, for it still partitions a whole person into discrete, fixable parts for remedying by a medical system. Even if a person were to check off all the seven components of WHO's health as "satisfactory," she may still be at a loss as to a larger story with which to guide her life's

---

25. Preamble to the Constitution of the World Health Organization as adopted by the International Health Conference, New York, June 19–22, 1946; signed on July 22, 1946 by the representatives of sixty-one states (Official Records of the World Health Organization, no. 2, p. 100) and entered into force on April 7, 1948 (www.who.int/about/definition/en/print/html). Since then the definition has been broadened to include as many as seven aspects of health: emotional, intellectual, physical, environmental, social, occupational, and spiritual.

26. McKenny, *To Relieve the Human Condition*.

27. Shuman, *Body of Compassion*, 84.

28. For an exploration of women's interactions with their bodies as "projects" see Brumberg, *Body Project*.

narrative. She could still be unhappy, even if she is "healthy" by WHO standards.

Health as a habit, then, doesn't save us, isn't higher than God or worthy of worship, nor is it conformity to science's understanding of health. Health as a habit isn't even the fluctuations in the way we feel from day to day or month to month, nor is it our genetic constitution. Rather, health as a habit constitutes our ethical intentions and efforts to live wholesome lives—lives that lead us deeper into love with God and our neighbor. Having explored fully what "habit" means and what "health" means, we can know see how the two function together.

Habit and Health: Running Together

This section affirms the agency present in "health as a habit." I'll work through the seven aspects of habit (habit as a lasting quality, oriented to action, repetitive, can increase/decrease/ is corruptible, constitutes virtue, is infused by God, has a telos to God) Aquinas offers in the treatise of habit, placing them in relationship to health. As a way of depicting how habit and health relate together to nudge someone toward wellbeing and relationship with God, I'll immerse the seven descriptions of habit into a case study of a person performing the healthy practice of long-distance running.

Habit as a Lasting Quality

Aquinas in affirms in I-II 49.1 that health does reside in the first species of quality, which indicates that as a habit it maintains a lasting consistency. Health, then, describes a body and soul orientation that is difficult to change.[29] Habits of health, like any other habit, are not easily lost and are well disposed in regards to something.[30]

---

29. Aquinas does indicate in *ST* I-II 50.1 that bodily dispositions are not difficult to change and are easily lost. This kind of health, which would include Aquinas's and his medical world's conceptions of the "humors," clearly refers to "health as a status" described earlier in the chapter. The fluctuating nature of the body is NOT the same thing as habits of health, which are stable and lasting. At the same time, the body does retain the capacity to nurture and sustain habit through the soul. For example, in I-II 50.1 Thomas states that habitual disposition can be in the body, compared to the soul as subject to form.

30. Aquinas, *ST* I-II 49.1.

PART ONE—Thomas Aquinas and Habits of Health

For example, a long distance runner (we'll call her Gena) exemplifies what it means to sustain health as a "lasting quality with consistency."[31] She gets up early almost every morning, puts on her running gear, and heads out the door to train. If she is out of town on a trip, or someone in her family needs her, or any multitude of life's circumstances intervene, she still finds a way to practice. Gena isn't easily dissuaded from running. For her running isn't just something to get done; this habit represents part of who she is. She says to others, "I am a runner." A habit that becomes quasi-permanent, that becomes like "second nature" (as Aquinas and Aristotle would say) describes a habit that has a lasting quality. For Gena running is such a habit.

Habit Orients to Action

Since habit implies an ordering to act, so too do virtuous practices of health. Aquinas quotes Aristotle in saying that a human being, or any part of his body can be considered healthy "when he can perform the operation of a healthy man."[32] Aristotle clarifies further that a habit of health "only makes us do healthy actions, not their contraries; for we say we are walking in a healthy way if [and only if] we are walking in the way a healthy person would."[33]

In the case of our runner Gena, her habit orients her to the healthy action of running. To be clear, the habit properly understood isn't the exercise itself, but the potentiality within her that inclines her to awaken before dawn, put on her shoes, and get moving. Gena's habit orients her to action, motivating her to move when natural forces (instinct) might

---

31. By using the example of running I'm not in any way wanting to diminish other dimensions of health. I'm simply focusing on a habit that I know well; before my MS-like attacks inhibited my gait and biomechanics, causing me eventually to hang up my running shoes, I was a competitive cross-country/distance runner from early adolescence into young adulthood. Gena was the captain of my cross-country team in high school when I was a freshman and sophomore. She taught me how to run with the passion of my heart and became my first close African-American friend; tragically in the spring of her senior year she died from an undetected congenital heart defect. I use her name as a way of upholding and remembering her virtuous practice of running.

32. Aristotle, *De Historia Animalium* X, I. 633b23–5 as quoted in Aquinas, *ST* I-II 49.3.

33. Arisotle, *Nicomachean Ethics* V, 1 (1129a). This obviously means that actions which inhibit or damage health can never be on a list of "healthy habits"—like smoking, excessive drinking, drug abuse, etc.

incline her to being sedentary (i.e., remaining in bed). Her movement, her action of engaging in the habit that sustains a running practice naturally leads to better health, because running demonstrates health.

Habit Bears Repeating

Habits of health require more than one action in order to be established within a person.[34] Health requires repeated, sustained effort.[35] In order to be a runner, for example, one must run over and over and over again—until it almost becomes natural and somewhat "easy" to run. Though the kinds of runs may vary each day (sprints, *fartleks*, hill training, etc) a runner must run often and repeatedly in order to maintain top conditioning. The more a runner runs the more she is transformed by her conditioning so that "good habits make us the types of persons who do good things readily."[36]

Habits Increase, Decrease, and Are Corruptible

Thomas recognizes that all of us come into the world differently; some of us receive robust constitutions and bodies, while others of us suffer endlessly with maladies and challenges.[37] "An equal degree of knowledge or health is received in one person more than in another because of a differing aptitude, either from nature or from custom."[38] Nonetheless, regardless of our "health as status" or how we were born into the world, we can cultivate habits to increase our health as part of an ongoing, lifelong moral pursuit in which we can realize increasing good even if we don't achieve the perfection of it.

---

34. Aquinas, *ST* I-II 51.2–3. For health, like in other habits, reason requires many repetitions in order for it to move the appetitive power enough for the memory to be impacted.

35. Ibid., I-II 51.

36. Mattison, *Introducing Moral Theology*, 59. Instead of running Mattison employs the example of repeatedly going to the gym in order to demonstrate how one acquires good habits.

37. Aquinas, *ST* I-II 51.1. "it may be natural according to the nature of the individual: as it is natural to Socrates or Plato to be sickly or healthy, each according to his own constitution."

38. Ibid., I-II 52.2.

PART ONE—Thomas Aquinas and Habits of Health

We increase habits of health just like any other habit—through our greater participation in the habit such that the habit produces a more perfect participation in its existing form.[39] In corporeal habits in particular, which would of course concern health, habit increases by intensity on behalf of the acting human being—an intensity that must display both interior desire and exterior potential.[40]

Our runner, Gena, easily exemplifies the phenomenon of habit increase. She decides to work more intensely with her coach over the next couple of months to train for an upcoming race. Under his guidance she does harder and faster speed intervals and adds more strength training to her routine. In just looking at the exterior results of her running, both her coach and she feel that her habit is increasing. Yet for her to be truly habituated into a stronger practice of running, Gina would have to have an "inner fire." She must not only do the difficult training runs, she must also desire in her heart to run harder and faster. Something about the pounding of her heart, the reach of her legs, the power of her billowing lungs—or even just the exhilaration when the run is over—must draw her. In order to be a champion athlete with greater intensity in training, Gina must love something about running. Her passion for the habit supports and sustains the actual action resulting from it. Gina's commitment to the habit is one of body and soul, of heart and mind, of inward and outward quality.

Yet suppose if for whatever reason her coach left her and she ceased training with the same level of intensity. In this scenario, Gina has only been conditioned into good shape; her training hasn't become a habit. She doesn't maintain any inward intensity without outward instigation. Her habit diminishes according to the different way she now participates in it.[41] Certainly her level of health diminishes along with that, from peak

---

39. Ibid., I-II 52.1-2. In I-II 52.2 Aquinas also states that we can talk about the habit itself as greater or lesser—"as health is said to be greater or less." He doesn't offer a specific example of a habit of health itself increasing.

40. Ibid., I-II 52.2. "That proportion, of course, which constitutes its health, may be brought to a more perfect state; but this comes about because of the change of simple qualities which admit only of that sort of change in intensive magnitude which concerns the degree to which their possessors possess them." In other words, the change in intensity would be far more the case for increase of habits of health than the change in the habit itself. However, Thomas does admit in the "reply to 1" on this question that bodily habit increase can still increase as itself—as by the addition of subject to subject.

41. Ibid., I-II 53.2. A habit "does diminish according to the different ways the subject participates in it." The demise of many well-intentioned diet/fitness plans after

athlete to recreational runner. Her habit must flow from who she is, from her internal character and passions, in order for her to sustain it. Without "fire" for what she is doing, her habit can only diminish—perhaps even to the point of ending completely.

The complete cessation, or corruption, of her habit of running (without any replacement exercise) would not only render her a disgruntled and possibly sick (or overweight) couch potato but would also mean she would stop observing the mean of health she once had. The existence of health's opposite of sickness means that health can be completely lost.[42] Without exercising her virtuous habit at all, she eventually loses it completely.[43] After months without running, were she to attempt to run around a track she would find herself panting and out of breath when once she could almost float across the pavement. Habits of health demand vigilant, balanced action or they and the health they sustain vanish.

Habits Constitute Virtue

Habits that dispose us to an act that is appropriate to our nature and conforms with reason are virtues. Since "health is a habit" and habits that dispose us to the good are virtues then it follows naturally to say that habits of health represent virtues.[44] Through habits of health we perform well and produce good.[45] In a similar way to which we must have inward and exterior intensity to match in order to maintain a habit, we must not only be adept at a habit of health, we must also direct its practice rightly toward the good.

Certainly aerobic fitness and strength comprises part of the healthy nature of a human being, so running (when practiced in the mean

---

their participants return home from a workshop weekend testifies to the presence of conditioning without habituation.

42. Aquinas, *Treatise on the Virtues*, I-II 53.1. "If therefore there should be some habit whose subject is corruptible and whose cause has a contrary, then the habit could be corrupted in either way, as is evident with bodily habits such as sickness and health."

43. Aquinas, *ST* I-II 53.3. "If a man does not exercise his virtuous disposition in moderating his feelings and actions, of necessity many feelings and actions will come about which will transcend the bounds of virtue, under the influence of the sense-appetite and other external pressures. And so his virtue will be lost, or weakened, if it is not exercised."

44. Ibid., I-II 49.2 and I-II 55.1.

45. Ibid., I-II 56.3.

without excess or deficiency), constitutes part of the "good" that is health. Consider again our runner Gena (who let's say has maintained her training and hasn't become a couch potato). Suppose she practices and trains diligently, and becomes quite good at running; she wins or comes close to winning the races she runs. However, if her running only becomes oriented to competition and winning, the moral goodness of her practice fades. Any virtue within her running completely erodes if she cheats or demonstrates unsportsmanlike conduct to others. Thus, she could be a really good runner without being "good" in the virtuous sense.

In order to be a good runner "inside and out," Gina must cultivate joy and dedication. She must run with an inner fire and an outer light. As she practices this habit of health, she becomes shaped by the endurance, character, diligence, and commitment required for long distance running. The habit of running improves more than her speed or resting heart rate; it enables her to become a more blessed person. Because she cultivates this habit she feels great physically and mentally, which enables her in turn to have more endurance and patience in order to serve God and her neighbor.

When we care for ourselves through habits of health, we become better people; such improvements are a part of Thomas's design for the virtuous life. Whether we run, or eat more vegetables, or take time to care for the health of our marriage, or seek out counseling during a time of grief, all of the habits of health we practice enable us to grow closer to God. Those things to which we dedicate time and energy in order to care for our embodied selves reap harvests not only of greater health, but more loving lives. As we become healthier we have greater capacity to worship God and tend to others. Taking time to practice a habit of health for ourselves remains the farthest thing from selfish or narcissistic; indeed nurturing a habit of health within us inevitably strengthens our ability to be faithful and to embody *caritas*.[46] Thomas's virtue ethic urges us to practice habits of health so that we might have the endurance and strength to live a true Christian life.

---

46. Habit's aspect of contributing to the lives of others is largely missing from secular programs for health, and according to Marie Griffiths in *Born Again Bodies*, historically most Christian health programs avoid any mention of service to neighbor.

Habits Can Be Infused by God

Aquinas thinks that God participates with us in the development of our habits of health. Once we have expended our efforts in a virtuous direction, God graciously strengthens whatever habit we have. Thomas names this strength imparted to us an infused habit—it has been infused with God's grace and represents one of the theological virtues of faith, hope and love. He writes that "acts produced by an infused habit do not cause a habit, but strengthen the habit already existing, just as medicinal treatment given to a man who is naturally healthy does not cause a healthy condition, but invigorates the health he already has."[47] Infused habits invigorate the habit we are already cultivating, giving us a gracious "boost" in order to sustain our healthy life of virtue.

For Gena, this means her habit of long distance running is sustained by grace. The gift of infused habit prevents her from relying completely upon her own efforts and exertions—a reliance which would represent a common Pelagianism within athleticism. Instead as she runs she can trust that the sustenance of her habit doesn't depend totally upon her. Perhaps Aquinas's understanding of infused habit really invites her to a place of trust. If she offers her body and soul to the increase of her habit, then she can rely on God's grace to keep her from failing. Though this gift doesn't extricate Gena from the responsibility for developing and sustaining her habits of health, grace does encourage her along the way to a more wholesome life.

Habits Have a Telos

Habits of health possess *teloi*. They lead persons to proximate ends. From the practice of a habit of health a person could lose weight, lower their blood pressure, gain fitness, reconcile with an estranged family member—the possibilities are endless. Each of these proximate ends are good; lower numbers on a blood pressure cuff or a weight scale would be celebrated by someone trying to lose weight.[48]

---

47. Aquinas, *ST* I-II 51.4.

48. However as proximate ends these results from the practices of health don't comprise the complete end of the story. In contrast, current weight loss programs (from Weight Watchers to the South Beach diet) and fitness regimes only maintain proximate ends. Nothing more exists for a practitioner than better scale numbers or greater levels of fitness.

PART ONE—Thomas Aquinas and Habits of Health

In Aquinas's moral schema though, the practices of health as proximate ends don't simply end there—health habits point to the larger end of friendship with God and support people along their way to that destination. When we practice habits of health with all the factors described above, we have greater energy, vitality, and strength so that we can worship God and love our neighbor. While not *eudaimonia* itself, habits of health nonetheless play an important role in ushering us along the path to happiness. Beatitude blesses us all the more when we can arrive at it without panting.

In Summation

Aquinas adopts, adapts, and elaborates upon Aristotelian philosophy of habit and health to develop his own moral strategy. Aquinas offers dual meanings of health that allow both for health to be a status, and a habit. Health as a status retains no moral component, and fluctuates dependent upon a person's heredity, immune system, and constitution. At the same time health can comprise part of a virtuous life as a person cultivates lasting habits in order to care for her wellbeing. We've also established what health is not for Aquinas, namely salvation, *summum bonum*, an idol, nor the WHO definition. Each of the seven aspects of habit—lasting quality, orients to action, repetitive, increases/decreases/is corruptible, constitutes virtue, is infused by God, has a telos—can be correlated to practices of health. The runner Gena serves as an example of such healthy habit cultivation. With a clear understanding of what is meant by habit and health, and the knowledge that health retains a moral significance in Aquinas, we can now move to consider more deeply the anthropology of habit, and how that impacts the unity of body and soul.

5

Body, Soul, and the Healthy Life

MATTERS OF HEALTH, THOUGH RANGING BEYOND THE HUMAN BODY, ARE also inextricable from the body. Habits that cultivate health necessarily, then, involve the whole person—body and soul. Aquinas, in his premodern and prenominalist understanding of the human person, portrays the body and soul as a unity, functioning in harmony together.[1] This holistic anthropology continues within the operations of the body and soul in habit. Aquinas's theological adeptness at maintaining the functions of soul and body in habit provides a foundation for health as a virtuous habit—since the body/soul remain inextricably interwoven with a person's experience of health. In other words, Aquinas's inclusion of the body (in union with the soul) as capable of habit affirms that practices of health can retain moral force.[2] In exploring below how Thomas attributes moral capacities to both the soul and the body, we'll perform a brief survey of the holism within Thomas's general anthropology, and then look specifically at the differentiation of habit into operative and entitative in the soul and the body. By uniting the body and soul in habits of health Thomas's anthropology promotes people's agency in tending to the wellbeing of their whole person. In the end, this holistic anthropology offers that bodies, just as much as souls, are for living a virtuous life oriented to God—a life that includes habits of health.

---

1. The advent of nominalism in the fourteenth century separated the human faculties from each other such that rationalism opposes voluntarism. This rupture led to Cartesian thought and the opposition of body to soul, science to tradition, and philosophy from theology. Suffice it to say here that Aquinas predates contemporary readers' rationalism and offers helpful, pre-nominalist perspectives on the human person.

2. Shuman, *Body of Compassion*, 119.

PART ONE—Thomas Aquinas and Habits of Health

Thomas's Holistic Anthropology

In Thomas's general anthropology three central concepts emerge that support the habituation of the body and adroitly avoid any hints of dualism found in Enlightenment thought. First, Thomas considers the human being a composite symphony of body and soul.³ "Body and soul are one being, one entity, absolutely speaking, not two entities."⁴ Each comprises part of the whole person, and separated out they cease to have the same meaning.⁵

Secondly, for Thomas the soul serves as the animating principle for the body.⁶ Thomas writes that:

> Therefore a body is competent to be a living thing or even a principle of life, as such a body. Now that it is actually such a body, it owes to some principle which is called its act. Therefore the soul, which is the first principle of life, is not a body, but the act of a body.⁷

As an animating form Thomas instead locates the soul within every part of the body and in no part at all.⁸ The soul gives life and action to the whole person.

Thirdly, Aquinas follows Aristotle in saying that soul is the *eidos*, or form of the body (*entelechy*), which comprises a single composite whole. He writes about the inseparable unity of soul and body in his commentary on Aristotle's *De Anima*:

> For, as is shown in the Metaphysics, Book VIII, form is directly related to matter as the actuality of matter; once matter actually is it is informed . . . therefore, just as the body gets its being from

---

3. Torrell, *Aquinas's Summa*, 32.

4. Klima, "Man=Body + Soul," 267. Klima notes that the root of philosophical problems about body and soul in Aquinas come from a post Cartesian assumption that the body and soul are two distinct entities of radically different natures.

5. Dillon, "As Soul to Body", 12. Aquinas states, for example, that a living (soul animated) body represents a different species than a dead, inanimate body. Aquinas, *ST* I-II 18.5.

6. Aquinas, *ST* 1.75.1. Aquinas offers a definition of the soul as the "first principle of life in those things which live."

7. Ibid.

8. Ibid., 1.76.3–5. Thomas is trying in these questions to deny any physical or corporeal nature of the soul.

the soul, as from its form so too it makes a unity with this soul to which it is immediately related.[9]

Aquinas's discussion of form and matter ultimately serves not to parse out the soul and body, but rather to affirm their integral unity as ensouled body, or embodied soul.[10] Taken together, these three features of Aquinas's anthropology (person as unity, soul as animating principle, and form/matter) supports an interdependent view of the body and soul in which both are required and both function together for the practice of habit and for the fullness of human life—in complete difference from the Cartesian severing of *res cognitans* from *res estensa*.

Yet even with this holistic anthropology, ambivalence exists in Thomas's treatment of the body in habit, in which he states in some places that there can be no habit in the body.[11] At the same time he argues that

9. Aquinas, *De Anima*, 2.1.234.
10. Dillon, "As Soul to Body," 16.
11. For an example of such ambivalence, in question fifty Aquinas states that the action of any body is attributable only either to natural powers or to the movement of the soul. Since natural powers, such as digestion in the body, have only one pathway for action (habits must necessarily be pluripotently disposed to action) the body's action from natural powers disqualifies it from habituation. Aquinas, *ST* I-II 50.1. As far as habit in the body from the movement of the soul goes the "body may be adapted and trained to minister promptly to the activities of the soul." This means that habit could be seen as marginally in the body only by reason of its ordering to the soul. Aquinas, *ST* I-II 50.2 Aquinas also writes in question 50.1 that the body is highly changeable because of the "mutability of physical causes"; the qualities of the soul, on the other hand, remain difficult to change. Therefore the body's easy alternation renders its qualities dispositions, rather than true habits. The body doesn't seem to be habitable from the perspective of question 50.1. In 50.3 Aquinas states further that "members of the body . . . have no habits, although there are habits of the faculties which command their movement." Aquinas, *ST* 50.3 Here Thomas makes a sophisticated argument that the appetitive sense powers that are acted upon by reason (not by natural instinct) can have habit within them; these same sense powers can then command the movement of the body. Thus it appears yet again that for Thomas the body doesn't possess habit. Lastly Aquinas argues in 55.2 that "human virtue . . . cannot belong to what is bodily, but only to what is proper to soul." Aquinas, *ST* I-II 55.2 He compares human bodies to nonrational animals and proclaims that it is only the rational powers of the soul that make humanity capable of habits of virtue. Again the body is excluded from participation in the practice of habits, while the soul, or the appetitive powers within the soul, can indeed participate in habituation. Yet, all these arguments delineated above that deny the body's primary participation in habit also seem to deny Aquinas's holistic anthropology described earlier. Rather than describing a human person as a unity of body and soul, I-II 50.1 seems to assert a hierarchy in which the soul directs the body to its commands. The soul appears to be not only the life principal but the only main actor in habituation. Instead of a description of form and matter as inextricable and

habit in the body functions secondarily as it is conditioned by the soul—seemingly giving a hierarchy to the function of habit in which the soul predominates.[12] In other articles he indicates that every activity of the human is a joint activity of soul and body and thus "no habit is in the soul alone but in the composite."[13] So how can we reconcile these seemingly contradictory notions of the role of the body in habit? If the body doesn't participate in habit at all, or even if habit comes to the body just because it hosts the soul, then we can't argue that health is a habit. Habit must be fully embodied in order for health to be considered part of the virtuous life.

Thomas himself provides a way out of this conundrum by differentiating how habit works in the body and the soul, while still maintaining his holistic anthropology. We'll look first at how operative habit functions in the soul, and then how entitative habit works in the body, to argue in the end that habit is indeed embodied, and thus health can be considered a vital part of the moral life—in contrast to the Cartesian dualist view in which morality cannot play a role in health.

---

indivisible, the above articles seem to denote a body easily separated out from the rationality of the soul. The composite unity of the human person and the possibility of the body carrying out habit would seem in doubt based upon this reading of I-II 50.1,3 and I-II 55. 1.

12. Aquinas, *ST* I-II 50. 1–2. In 50.1 Thomas affirms that habit can be in the body, since the form of the soul can only exist in the matter of the human body—but here again habit exists in the body only by connection to the soul. Anthony Kenny, "appendix 8" in Aquinas, *ST*, 125.

13. Aristotle *De Anima* 1 (403a 8); 4 (408b 8) quoted in Aquinas, *Treatise on the Virtues*, I-II 50. 4.

A Tale of Different Habits I: Operative Habits and the Soul[14]

Aquinas clearly thinks that the soul cultivates habit because it (the soul) is pluripotent, directs action, and its qualities are difficult to change.[15] Aquinas develops the notion of habit in the soul by describing it as operative; "it is through its faculties (Latin-*potentias* or powers) that the soul is the source of activities (Latin- *operationum* or operations), habits of this kind are habits of the faculties (*potentias*- powers)."[16] Said another way, the powers of the soul activate habit, and that habit is operative.[17]

---

14. I am grateful to Dr. Reinhard Huetter for a conversation in which he delineated the differences of operative and entitative habits. While Thomas himself doesn't use the terms "entitative" or "operative" the substance of the distinction is present in the Summa, later Thomist interpreters developed these designations in order to name a distinction that runs throughout the whole treatise on habit (I-II q.49-54) in the *Summa* and is most specifically named in I-II 49.3, responsio 3. Here Thomas states that "every habit is in some way connected with action . . . but the nature of a thing is itself directed to another goal, which is either action, or the product of an action. So a habit is connected not only with the nature [entitative] of its possessor, but also, in consequence, with an action [operative]." See also for this distinction: ST I-II, 50, 1: "Habit is a disposition of a subject which is in a state of potentiality either to form [nature] or to operation."

ST I-II, 50, 2: "Habit implies a certain disposition in relation to nature or to operation."

ST I-II, 54, 1: "Habits are dispositions of a thing that is in potentiality to something, either to nature, or to operation, which is the end of nature." Dr. Huetter described the distinction this way: "Entitative habits" denote the modification of a substance in relation to its being and form (body), while operative habits modify the operative powers (soul) of a substance. Wherever Thomas, in the treatise on habit, talks about certain dispositions in relation to nature, his later interpreters use the term "entitative habits" because they qualify the nature of the substance; wherever he talks about dispositions in relation to operation, his interpreters use the term "operative habits" because these habits qualify the operative powers of the substance.

15. Aquinas, *ST* I-II 50.2. Pluripotency is required in the definition of habit. It should also be explained that Aquinas follows Aristotle in having vegetative, sensitive, and intellectual aspects of the soul. The vegetative wouldn't be seen as having habit primarily because of its lack of dependency on reason. In Aquinas, *ST* I-II 50.1 he cites Aristotle, *Nicomachean Ethics* II, 1 (1103b21), describing habit as oriented to action. In Aquinas, *ST* I-II 50.1 Thomas indicates that habits in the soul are difficult to change.

16. Aquinas, *ST* I-II 50.2. I offer the Latin here because I believe it renders the sense of "operative habit" better than Kenny's translation.

17. Aquinas restates this also in Aquinas, *Treatise on the Virtues*, I-II 51.2. "Habit is a disposition for operation, whose subject is the power of the soul." However, the essential powers of the soul (sense appetite, intellect, and will) don't suffice for a person to initiate action; these powers must be oriented by the first species of quality, known as habit.

The operative habits of the soul lead a person to virtue: "human virtue does not imply relation to being, but rather to activity. Essentially, then, it is an operative habit."[18] The "potency for action" in the soul with rational powers disposes people to flourishing and the end of friendship with God.[19] Without a doubt then, the operative habits within the soul enable someone to practice habits that include health and to obtain the end of *eudaimonia*. This ability to practice health and live into flourishing differs dramatically from the passivity inculcated into people from a dualist perspective of body and soul. For Aquinas our souls grant us the ability to live better lives; for Descartes souls confer upon us the ability to think and reason. Obviously then, operative habits lead to health in ways that the *res cognitans* simply cannot.

A Tale of Different Habits II: Entitative Habit and the Body

Aquinas believes that more habits exist than just operative ones (ordered to an action in the soul) within a human being.[20] He states that there can be different kinds of habits within one passive power: "Many habits can be in one power. And just as there are many genera in one genus, and many species in one species, so there may be various species of habits and of power."[21] The second kind of habit, also called entitative, orders to a nature instead of an action. It indicates a relatively permanent (remembering that habit cannot readily change) substance of a being, and is thus oriented to matter and the body.[22]

---

18. Aquinas, *ST* I-II 55.2. In the Blackfriars edition of volume 23 (questions 55–67) W. D. Hughes does translate *operativus* as "operation" rather than "activity" (as did Kenny). It should be noted that a typing error appears in the paperback Blackfriars edition, labeling article two as article one—when it is in fact article two. See also Aquinas, *ST* I-II 50.1 in which Aquinas indicates that a habit is disposed either to form (entitative) or activity (operative habit).

19. Aquinas, *ST* I-II 55.2

20. Ibid., I-II 54.1. "there are many habits in a single subject."

21. Aquinas, *Treatise on the Virtues*, I-II 54.1. I prefer Oesterle's translation of this passage for its clarity.

22. Aquinas, *ST* I-II 55.2. "Man is so constituted that his body is like matter, his soul like form. As for the body, that indeed a man possesses in common with other animals, and likewise the powers common to animated body." Aquinas, *Treatise on the Virtues*, 67 n. 4. However, since entitative habit is not directed by the rational power of the soul, it isn't capable of supernatural ends. Instead, entitative habits can achieve

Aquinas can also say without contradiction that habit cannot be in the body when it moves only by natural qualities; the movements of digestion, for example, are not directed by any operative or entitative habit because they have the potentiality for only one act.[23] These bodily functions (digestion, excretion, breath, heartbeat, etc.) occur without any conscious direction on a human being's part; thus Thomas considered them part of the vegetative soul. Bodily functions, which for Aquinas are without habit, are to be distinguished from the nature of the body, which can be conditioned by entitative habit—this distinction explains how Aquinas can say both that habit is not/is in the body.[24]

For Aquinas entitative habit in the body can have natural beginnings: "there are some rudimentary appetitive habits which are natural to individuals on account of their bodies. Some people, for instance, are disposed by their bodily constitution to chastity, others to mildness of temper, and so on."[25] In other cases entitative habits result from conditioning within the body. These conditioned entitative habits must be moved by the operative habits of the soul.[26] "There can be a habit of the body adapted to the soul, there cannot be a habit of the soul adapted to the body."[27] The "being" habit of entitative requires the power of operative habit in order to execute to its object.

However, entitative habit's orientation to operative doesn't mean that the soul directs the body in an authoritative, hierarchical manner. Aquinas cites Aristotle to indicate that the habits of the body and soul (entitative and operative) function to the best accord for their nature.[28] This joint functioning is "an activity of the whole person" such that "it follows that any habit belongs not to the soul alone but to the person as

---

proximate ends; proximate ends constitute goods, just simply not ultimate goods.

23. Aquinas, *ST* I-II 50.1.

24. However one could also argue that even bodily functions could be improved by good entitative habits. The conditioning of the body through good diet and exercise, for example, would improve digestion. Modern science has shown that our physical organs contain receptor sites for neurochemicals of thought and emotion and can even manufacture some of these themselves; thus reason is located throughout the body and not just in the brain or "soul." Our knowledge of anatomy over Aquinas's day means that even natural functions could be connected to the entitative habits of the body.

25. Aquinas *ST* I-II 51.1.

26. Ibid., I-II 50.1–2.

27. Ibid., I-II 50. 2.

28. Ibid., I-II 49.2 quoting Aristotle, *Physics* VII , 3 (246a 13).

a whole."²⁹ This holistic understanding of habit means that the soul and body move together in a harmonious dance toward a life of virtue; one isn't higher or authoritarian over the other.

The conditioning of the body through entitative habit as directed by the operative habit of the soul resembles a trained ballet dancer.³⁰ Through days, weeks, months, and years of practice at the barre and repetition of steps her body is conditioned through entitative habit. Her legs develop muscle and her arms tone as she practices; her body reveals entitative habit even as her soul moves her to dedication to her craft. The dance of entitative and operative habit in the body and soul affirms Aquinas's holistic anthropology. Both function in unity as matter and form duet together to direct the person to a life of virtue.

The understanding of entitative and operative habits described above means that the body is capable of habituation. While some aspects of the body can easily fluctuate (with a cold/flu, with a dinner of too many sweets, etc.) the entitative habits that function with the body are not as easily changeable; for example a ballet dancer of many years doesn't easily loss her passion for training or her ability to sharply point her foot or do a *jete*.

Aquinas also makes the connection that the body's disposition through habit orients it toward health.³¹ A person practicing good entitative habits in the body (as directed by the soul) arrives at greater health and beauty than she would without such habits.³² Health serves as a proximate end for entitative habits. In fact, if one is cultivating virtuous entitative habits, one can't help but sustain a body oriented to a healthier life. In sum, Thomas's holistic anthropology, instilled in habit through his understanding of the operative and entitative, empowers people to cultivate healthier lives in soul and body. This holism in soul and body extends to our emotional health as well, which Thomas terms the passions. To these passions we turn in the next chapter.

---

29. Ibid., I-II 50.4 citing Aristotle, *De Anima* I, 1 (403a 8); (408b 8).

30. Ibid., I-II 50.2 describes the movement of the body by the soul.

31. Ibid., I-II 54.1. Klubertanz also indicates that health is an entitative habit. Klubertanz, *Habits and Virtues*, 98 n. 22.

32. Aquinas, *ST* I-II 55.2. "Virtue, as being a fitting disposition of soul, is likened to health and beauty, which are fitting dispositions of body."

6

Passionately Longing for Health

DUE TO THOMAS'S HOLISTIC ANTHROPOLOGY, NOT ONLY DOES HE INCLUDE the body and soul in his conception of habits of health, he also includes the passions. Aquinas believes we maintain responsibility over how we feel about situations, which means our emotions partake in the moral life—a moral life that includes health, as argued above.[1] As a "movement of the sensitive appetite" reason guides the passions to either good or evil.[2] For Aquinas emotions can certainly serve the good of directing us closer to God, the source of all that completes us.[3] For Thomas we are creatures of passions and appetites because we experience so deeply our incompleteness: "a human being is one whose very nature is appetite, whose whole being is a turning toward all those goods which promise fullness of life."[4] Thomas understood this passion and based his moral system around it; we, who dwell in the universe of God's gracious

---

1. Cates, *Choosing to Feel*, 13. Cates cites Aristotle's *Nicomachean Ethics* (1102b30–32) and (1114a3–11).

2. Aquinas, *ST* I-II 59.1. Oesterle in Aquinas, *Treatise on the Virtues* I-II 59.1 footnote 2 describes passions as emotions. White, "The Passions of the Soul," 106. Aquinas follows the Peripatetic view here that passions are an important part of the moral life and are neither good or bad, but are more perfect when moderated by reason. Aquinas states that "the passions, considered in themselves, can go both to good and evil, according as they can agree or be at odds with reason." Aquinas, *ST* I-II 59.1. Aquinas delineates the passions into concupisciple (love, desire, joy, hatred, aversion, sorrow) and the irascible (hope, despair, fear, courage, anger). Aquinas, *ST* I-II 60.4.

3 Miner, *Thomas Aquinas on the Passions*, 92. Miner notes that Aquinas, the laconic master of understatement, affirms that passions perfect human good five times, which underscores the importance of the emotions in the moral life for him. He also expands Aristotle's definition by understanding the passions as directed ultimately to God. Mattison, *Introducing Moral Theology*, 81. Passions aren't blind surges of feeling, but are intelligible and reasonably guided responses to types of situations.

4. Wadell, *Primacy of Love*, 81.

love, long to return that love back to the divine source by loving others and by being loved.[5] Inevitably then, the greater we grow in love through passions oriented to God, the healthier we become; a life of emotions directed rightly represents a life lived in balance and harmony—by all means a healthier life.

Thomas recognized that our feelings, our passions—our deepest desire to be loved and to love--comprise an essential part of the virtuous life because it's only when we care enough about something that we do anything; as humans we have to feel in order to act.[6] When we fervently devote ourselves to loving God through our passions, we consequently experience greater wholeness and healing in our lives. In this next section we will explore in greater depth the connection between our passions, the virtuous life, and our embodied experience of wellbeing with God.

The Passions' Relationship to Virtue

Passions are essential to the moral life; "the moral virtues, which are about passions as their proper matter, cannot be without the passions."[7] "Those moral virtues which are concerned with passions as their proper matter cannot exist apart from them."[8] In the case of health, for example, we have to be passionate enough about our wellbeing in order to lend any moral effort to its maintenance. For the gift of life God has given to us, God demands our highest ardor (passion) in order that we might attain the greatest health we may have through good habits.[9]

---

5 Wadell, *Primacy of Love*, 83. Wadell describes us as acting to love because it has first acted upon us. Said another way "the goodness of life thrusts itself through and leaves its mark on our souls."

6. Ibid., 79.

7. Aquinas, *Treatise on the Virtues*, I-II 59.5. Wadell, *Primacy of Love*, 90. Aquinas, *ST* I-II 59.1. Aquinas states that moral virtue cannot be a passion, but rather is a principle of the appetite's movement. While not all moral virtues concern themselves with passions—some are about operations—moral virtues are not without their passions. Aquinas, *ST* I-II 59.4.

8. Aquinas, *ST* I-II 59.5 Aquinas quotes Aristotle to indicate that passions are consequent to acts of virtues. "the Philosopher says . . . "if virtues are about actions and passions, and delight and sorrow follow upon every action and every passion, then by reason of this, virtue will be concerned with delight and sorrow." Aquinas, I-II 59.4 quoting Aristotle, *Nicomachean Ethics*, II 3 (1104b 13–15).

9. Barth, *The Doctrine of Creation*, 357. Barth makes the point that even healthy people always maintain the risk of losing their health and run a greater risk of negligence of their health—which could result in them becoming more incapacitated than

Habits, including habits of health, function in the life of virtue to qualify the passions. Habit conditions not only what we *do* for our health but also how we *feel* about our health. They "instill intelligence in emotions" by disciplining and controlling the vicissitudes of our feelings.[10] Habit names the possibility of responsibility for our emotional life.[11] In other words, through habit we condition ourselves not only with how we act, but also with how we feel.[12] The moral challenge of the passions is not to repress them, but rather to order them properly to the good.[13] A runner, for example, may not feel like braving a hot, humid summer's morning, but her disciplined habit shapes her emotions so that she decides to put on her running shoes anyway. After a mile of running her emotions are gladdened and she renews her passionate devotion to her practice of health—a practice through which she deepens her relationship with God. For Aquinas, even raw or spontaneous emotion (like disgust at horrible, hot weather) can governed and schooled by a life of reasoned morality toward the end of greater love of God.[14]

The passions at work in habits of health, then, rightly orient us to friendship with God. By our emotions drawing us into deeper devotion to our practices of health, we are pulled into greater zeal for the goodness of God. God at work through our passions draws us to the source of love that heals and makes us whole.[15]

---

those whom know who have chronic disease conditions. He writes, "He (the healthy person) may be severely handicapped in the exercise of this power, and therefore sick, long before this makes itself felt in the deterioration of his organs or their functional disturbance, so that he perhaps stands in greater need of the summons that he should be healthy than someone who already suffers from such deterioration and disturbance and is therefore regarded as sick in soul or body or perhaps both."

10. Titus, *Resilience and the Virtue of Fortitude*, 116.
11. Dunnington, "Addiction and Action," 50.
12. Cates, *Choosing to Feel*, 27.
13. Pope, "Overview of the Ethics of Thomas Aquinas," 33.
14. Miner, *Thomas Aquinas on the Passions*, 97. White, "The Passions of the Soul," 45-46. "For Aquinas, events within the soul produce distinct bodily events. But the distinction is not a separation. Because the body and soul are fundamentally integrated, there will always be an ordered connection between them."
15. Wadell, *Primacy of Love*, 92.

PART ONE—Thomas Aquinas and Habits of Health

Embodied/Ensouled Passion

The healing and wholeness at work in the passions involves both the composite of body and the soul—especially since habit (as we have shown above) involves both.[16] In humans the will, or appetitive power, approves the passion that is then carried out within the body.[17] In this performance the body isn't slavish to the will, but functions as a free agent in which it can resist (or obey) reason's direction within the soul.[18] This unitive functioning of the soul and body in the performance of passions not only resists Cartesian dualism, but also affirms a person's whole-self passionate involvement in the care of their health.

For example, sorrow as a passion necessarily involves the body and the soul. Thomas spends the most time (five questions) on the emotion of sorrow; when we suffer both body and soul are inextricably impacted.[19] When we grieve, we feel grief not just emotionally, but through weary, exhausted bodies that crave sleep and souls that are forlorn.[20] In such an experience of loss, habits that would sustain health in the midst of the passion of sorrow might include communal worship (particularly a memorial service) and the maintenance of good nutrition; in order to perform these habits a person must desire with her whole being to continue living fully even in the midst of grief.

More recent research into psychosomatic unity indicates that what we feel impacts our body and in turn, our health, in complex interrelated ways—affirming Thomas's understanding of the embodied/ensouled relationship of passion and habit.[21] Aquinas's thought on the body and

---

16. Miner, *Thomas Aquinas on the Passions*, 32. White, "The Passions of the Soul."

17. White, "The Passions of the Soul," 105. Other animals carry out the bodily experience of passion without any direction from the rational will.

18. Ibid., 45–46.

19. Miner, *Thomas Aquinas on the Passions*, 188, 202, 206. Thomas considers sorrow a passion that can deepen the soul and prepare it for the gift of true humility. He does feel that immoderate sorrow can harm the body and lead to *acedia*. He offers that sleep and baths can help to mitigate the effects of sorrow.

20. Cates, *Choosing to Feel*, 25. Cates gives an extended example of how her experience of bodily commotion points to passions at work. She writes, "we can only perceive well what is required of us morally if we perceive with passion appropriate to the situation in which we find ourselves, that is, if we grasp relevant features of the situation in an embodied, desire-full way."

21. However, Thomas's indication in *ST* I-II 50.3 (reply to 3) that the bodily members have no habits in them is no longer supportable by contemporary accounts of the interrelationship of the passions and the body. Aquinas, *ST* I-II 50.3 translated

soul as functioning in unity in the passions means that good habits of health can direct our emotions. Our inner desires for wholeness express themselves through our entire person, body and soul, urging us onward to the healing life of virtue with God.

Passionate for Health

If we are to yearn with all of our passions for health as a good from God, how are those not "born well" or who suffer with debilitating chronic diseases to seek for health? How can their passion for wellbeing possibly be satisfied if they always remain sick or disabled? Is Thomas right then when he indicates that one can't be healthy unless "all of its parts are healthy and beautiful?"[22] Must all of these people who already endure so much through their bodies have to endure even longer until the eschaton when their health can finally be in "perfect proportion?"[23]

Karl Barth provides helpful guidance to these questions when he writes:

> Sickness is obviously negative in relation to health ... It hinders man in his exercise of them by burdening, hindering, troubling and threatening him, and causing him pain. But sickness as such is not necessarily impotence to be as man. The strength to be this, so long as one is still alive, can also be the strength and therefore the health of the sick person. And if health is the strength for human existence, even those who are seriously ill can will to be healthy without any optimism or illusions regarding their condition. They too are commanded, and it is not too much to ask, that so long as they are alive they should will this, i.e. exercise the power that remains to them, in spite of every obstacle. Hence it seems to be a fundamental demand of the ethics of the sick bed that the sick person should not cease to let himself be addressed, and to address himself, in terms of health and the will which it requires rather than sickness, and above all to see to it that his is in an environment of health.[24]

---

by Anthony Kenny, footnote g, 36–37. Here Thomas isn't refuting the possibility of entitative habit in the whole body, but rather remarking on different parts of the body. Kenny notes that, contrary to what Aquinas asserts, the eye or the palate could be trained—indicating that habits (namely entitative habits) can be in the body.

22. Aquinas, *ST* I-II 52.3.
23. Ibid.
24. Barth, *Doctrine of Creation*, 357–58.

PART ONE—Thomas Aquinas and Habits of Health

While affirming the reality and challenges of sickness, Barth nonetheless teaches that in every way the virtuous life demands sick people to pursue health.[25] Through the exercise of whatever strength they possess, they insist on living and retain the dignity of their personhood. By exercising the faculties of body or soul that they have, sick people refuse to capitulate to the powers of death—powers that are opposed to the good will of God as Creator.[26] The pursuit of health in the midst of disability or disease with the dedication of one's passions doesn't represent folly, but rather a faithful following of the Christ who overcame the chaos and death such maladies represent.[27]

When a person with a chronic disease dedicates herself to eating a strict diet that supports her health, or sacrifices time and money in order to train at the gym, she affirms her own life as gift. When she perseveres through incessant pain or dedicates herself to seeking healers that can help her, she participates in God's desire for her to have health. While her passion for health must remain in the mean (her pursuit of health ceases to be virtuous if she becomes so obsessed by it she stops worshipping God and worships health instead), the passionate yearning to be healthy comprises an invaluable part of the virtuous life. Barth affirms the moral significance of passionately desiring for health when he writes:

> Human willing and acting with God, and in orientation on Him, and with faith and prayer to Him, whatever the outcome, has the promise which man cannot lack, and the fulfillment of which he will soon see, if he will simply obey without speculation. Those who take up this struggle obediently are already healthy in the fact that they do so, and theirs is no empty desire when they will to maintain or regain their health.[28]

Therefore, those who are diseased or disabled can attain health through their passionate struggle to be healthy.[29] Our embodied/

---

25. Ibid., 364. Barth notes that illness is not an illusion (though hypochondriacs do exist!).

26. Ibid., 367.

27. Ibid., 366.

28. Ibid., 369.

29. Aquinas perhaps gets it wrong then, when he suggests that all the parts of a person must be healthy in order for her to be called healthy. Aquinas, ST I-II 52.2. However, he also states in I-II 52.2 that health can vary, and is susceptible to more or less while the person can still be called healthy. This discrepancy in Thomas may be due to a difference between health as status and health as entitative habit, or could also be ambivalence in the text.

ensouled passion for health expressed through habit, even in the midst of disease, urges us onward toward greater wellbeing and deeper love of God. Thomas's understanding of the passions affirms that we are creatures who must feel and then act; the actions that come out our yearnings lead to virtuous habits that form us into more vibrant, healthier human beings who are falling deeper into love with our Creator.

7

The Action of Habits of Health

HAVING ESTABLISHED THAT HABITS OF HEALTH NECESSARILY INCLUDE the body, the soul, and the passions we now move to the action of habits of health. This section offers an answer to the questions, "How does habit actually work? How would someone wanting to cultivate a healthier life begin to practice a new habit?" In order to answer these questions we'll first examine Thomas's understanding of action's development through the will, reason, and habit. We'll then place this Thomist development of habit within the contemporary work of psychologists Prochaska, Norcross, and DiClemente on stages of change. By intersecting Aquinas's wisdom with the psychologists' model we can provide a clear pathway for how someone might begin a new virtuous habit of health. The practice of running will serve as an example of new habit cultivation. Through this section's discussion of action we'll depict how someone actually does employ their agency to make changes in their life through healthy habits. These transformations certainly support a virtue-based care of health in which a person nurtures the excellence of his mind, body, spirit, and emotions through habit.

The Action of Habit in Aquinas

Thomas's understanding of how habit works in the person is one of fluidity in motion—like a great dance in which one step flows into the next and sometimes may even repeat itself before the dance comes to its completion. In this dance Aquinas is mainly concerned with moral virtue (though he does acknowledge that the intellect can be the subject of virtue).[1] These habits of moral virtue move with the appetitive powers.[2]

However, habits' "dance" with the powers is not comprised of simple steps (1, 2, 3); Thomas's understanding of the action of habit becomes an argument in how difficult it is to be good. Thomas notes that the development of good habits often must overcome vicious habits; such uprooting remains challenging because of the power of vice.[3] A beginner must first work diligently to overcome the vices and their moral life becomes one of healing from chronic woundedness. The novice then moves to establish the virtues more strongly within her as she participates more strongly in the goodness of God. Lastly, she develops into a virtuous person who enjoys God and is good as God is good.[4] In the following discussion of how habit moves in the person, we'll assume vice is overcome—at least enough to allow for the "dance" of good habits to begin. The main partners in this "dance" are the will, reason, and habit itself, all of which affirm that the human person acts as a moral agent for her health.

The Will

The will names the power of the soul as ordered by reason through which a human being is in control of her actions.[5] Said another way the will is the power by which a person directs her actions to the good—the will

---

1. Aquinas, *ST* I-II 56.3 "Hence the intellect also, inasmuch as it is subordinate to the will, can be the subject of virtue in its unqualified sense. In this way the speculative intellect or reason is the seat of faith; for the intellect is moved by the command of the will to assent to what is of faith, since no man believes unless he is willing. The practical intellect, on the other hand, is the seat of prudence." The speculative intellect confers an aptitude for truth, and the practical intellect confers prudence. Aquinas, *ST* I-II 57.1. However, virtue induces not only the aptitude to act well (which the intellect can do) but also the right use of action (which the intellect cannot do). Aquinas, *ST* I-II 56.3

2. Ibid., I-II 57.1

3. Ibid., I-II 51.3. Here Thomas argues that it takes more than one act of virtue to establish a habit, indicating the perseverance required to overcome vice. Vice can also be habitual and can discourage us from our efforts to try and be good. Aquinas, *ST* II-II 24.9.

4. Wadell, *Primacy of Love*, 120. Wadell asserts that one never fully "arrives"—we are always journeying to be more virtuous; there is no limit to the virtues' growth within us. He also describes this journey from beginner to practitioner to expert as the three stages of acquiring virtue in Thomas.

5. Gallagher, "The Will and Its Acts," 69–70.

ensures that a person can indeed inscribe herself into good practices.[6] For Thomas the will is both mover and moved (in this section the will is discussed as "mover"; in the section below on habit it becomes "the moved"). As a mover it enables a person to act well: "that a man actually acts well is because he has a good will. Consequently, the virtue which actually makes him to act well, and not merely to be capable of doing so, must be either in the will itself, or in some power as moved by the will."[7]

For example, in regards to health a person could orient his will toward better food choices. By choosing food grown in harmony with the earth (organically, biodynamically, on a small local farm) he aligns his will not only with what promotes health, but also with how God created us to eat (i.e. not from an industrialized food machine). By directing his eating habits toward the good, the person lives into God's will and acts well for his own moral life and health.

However, the will, or the power exercised through deliberative action, doesn't easily move to what a person might want (even if it is healthy food). The movement of the will demands intense concentration and discipline and taxes the person. It cannot sustain itself on its own.[8] The will is a human power that needs to be disciplined in one direction so that it isn't subject to corruption or alteration. The will can only initiate the act in moral virtue and move reason to its object; it requires habit in order to keep it disciplined.[9]

Reason

Reason's object is habit. By repeated acts of the will acting upon reason and that reason in turn acting, "a certain quality is produced in the passive potentiality which is acted upon, and it is this quality which is called a habit."[10] Habit builds in its potential power such that it is disposed and

---

6. Ibid., 73.

7. Aquinas, *ST* I-II 56.3. The will requires the coordination of a number of powers and is quite complex. Aquinas goes on to say that the intellect, or reason, is moved by the will; a person turns his mind (intellect) to something because he wills to do so.

8. Dunnington, "Addiction and Action," 40.

9. Aquinas, *ST* I-II 50.1. This movement of the will proceeds "from the soul through the body." Though rooted in the soul, the will is constrained and disciplined by the body. This means that the exercise of the will requires the body for its full execution and movement to its object; the body remains significant in the very beginnings of an act. So for Aquinas, even the action of the will remains holistic—in the body and soul.

10. Ibid., I-II 51.2.

ordered to action, but doesn't consist of action in and of itself.[11] Reason constitutes the active principle here.[12]

As the active principle, reason can guide a person toward better actions for their health. A man trying to choose between an apple and Apple Jacks (a processed cereal) can utilize reason to sway his decision toward the good; for example, the man reasons that the cereal is full of sugar, was completely manufactured, and contributes to obesity, whereas the apple is a part of creation and full of easily digested fructose energy. By actively reasoning between two options and choosing what is better, the person orients toward the health God would have for him. Such reasoning for Aquinas isn't about control; instead the reason involved in virtuous habits of health orients to flourishing.

Habit

The will, as described above, must have within it inclining qualities called habits, which moves the appetitive power to its object. Here the will is nudged, or inclined by habit; it is the "moved."[13] Habit inclines the will to a good determined by reason in order that action can promptly follow.[14] Habit, in other words, guides the will to choose rightly.[15] *Habitus* names the possibility of acting well without requiring constant and exhausting vigilance from the will.[16] It explains how the will can act without being eroded or worn down; it sustains the will in acting consistently amidst a myriad of desires and options by qualifying and coordinating desires.[17]

---

11. Ibid., I-II 54.1. "It is only passive faculties which are subjects of habits: a faculty which is purely active is not the subject of any habit."

12. Ibid., I-II 51.3.

13. Ibid., I-II 50.5. "The will is both mover and moved" from Aristotle *De Anima* III, 10 (433b 16).

14. Ibid.

15. Kent, "Habits and Virtues," 119. Here Aquinas departs from Aristotle in saying that habit is principally related to the will. Aristotle holds people responsible for action even when they act against their own choice or reasoned conception of the good. For Aquinas we never act from passion without the consent of our wills.

16. Dunnington, "Addiction and Action," 40.

17. Ibid., 43. It is important to note here that habit is not equivalent to instinct. It is like instinct in that it makes an action easy and seemingly effortless. However habit responds to the work of reason, whereas instinct is imbedded within a creature's nature and is not responsive to reason. Dunnington, "Addiction and Action," 46.

These habits, which orient the will and are nudged into potentiality from reason, dwell within the appetitive powers.[18] Habit is actually in the human nature prior to the power as potentiality.[19] The appetitive powers (or sensory powers), as moved by reason and inclined by habit, then move to act.[20]

The end result of an action that supports virtue comes from the complex interaction of will, reason, habit, and appetitive powers. This intricate dance isn't linear and can't easily be diagrammed; instead the whole body and soul work together to shape a virtuous person. "It is natural for the soul to be united to the body. . . the perfection of the soul cannot exclude the natural perfection of the body."[21] Aquinas understands that the perfecting process for good virtues to be fostered through action can be a long journey.[22] Yet Thomas believes that the action of habit within us can cultivate embodied, ensouled virtues that transform us. Thomas's thought on the action of habit empowers each person so that through their own agency (will, reason, and habit) they can engage in practices that promote flourishing—enabling them to be fully alive and in service to others.

Habits of Health and the Work of Change

Habits of health would function in the same way as the "dance" described above: the will acts upon reason, which in turn acts to produce a "passive potentiality" known as a habit. The habit then moves the will, or appetitive power, to consistently achieve its object without being eroded or worn down. However, Aquinas's understanding of the nature of action in habit might seem esoteric and inaccessible. By pairing Aquinas's thought on the will, reason, and habit with an easily comprehensible psychological

---

18. Ibid., 49. Habits aren't completely determined by the process of deliberative reason from the will. Instead they are "like a second nature" and consist of patterned acts that aren't fully willed through reason, nor fully automatic or instinctual.

19. Aquinas, *ST* I-II 50. 2

20. Ibid., I-II 51.2.

21. Aquinas, *Treatise on Happiness*, 49.

22. Wadell, *Primacy of Love*, 118. Aquinas understood this journey as having three major stages: 1. The virtues of beginners, in which the virtue is working to overcome vice 2. Virtues of those on their way, in which they are practicing goodness 3. Virtues of those who have arrived, in which they are enjoying life with God.

text on stages of change, a practical way of thinking through how a person might actually begin to cultivate a new habit of health emerges.

Contemporary psychologists and professors James Prochaska, John C. Norcross, and Carlo DiClemente offer in their book *Changing For Good: A Revolutionary Six-Stage Program For Overcoming Bad Habits and Moving Your Life Positively Forward* a straightforward account of how people might begin new healthy habits or change bad ones. These psychologists delineate stages of change (precontemplation, contemplation, preparation, action, maintenance, and termination) that human beings progress through in order to make lasting alterations to their lives. Certainly *Changing For Good* lacks any larger *telos* beyond the change itself and it focuses much more upon eradicating bad habits rather than cultivating good ones. They don't explicitly reference Aquinas nor virtue ethics--theirs is a secular, psychological text. Nonetheless their strategies for change are amenable to an account of habit and can elucidate how a person might actually begin to practice a habit of health.[23] Below I will utilize Prochaska, Norcross, and DiClemente's stages of change (minus termination) in order to describe the development of a habit of health—in this case running.[24] In this model a person must know which stage they are in order for the change to be effective; by knowing their stage a person can take appropriate action at the right time.[25]

---

23. Other modern psychologists have given us accounts that focus upon habit, including people such as William James, Charles Pierce, John Dewey, and George Klubertanz. I chose Prochaska, Norcross, and DiClemente's work because it elucidates a clear and practical model of behavior change that is amendable to Aquinas's understanding of habit.

24. I leave out their stage of termination because in Aquinas's model, we always want to maintain good habits of health, while their model is mainly concerned with the cessation of bad habits.

25. Prochaska, Norcross, DiClemente, *Changing For Good*, 15. The authors spend an entire chapter describing the psychological processes of how people change—through consciousness raising, social liberation, emotional arousal, self-reevaluation, commitment, countering, environmental control, rewards, and helping relationships. All of these processes have their origins in diverse schools of psychotherapy; the authors concur that many of these could be applied in different ways in order to effect change. I refrain from more explicit application of such techniques in a discussion of habit because that would lead down the path to casuistry in ethics, which Thomas assiduously avoids.

PART ONE—Thomas Aquinas and Habits of Health

Precontemplation

People at this first stage have no intention of changing their behavior and usually deny that they should adopt any new habits (or drop problematic ones). Often demoralized, they lack the willpower to make a difference in their own life.[26] For Aquinas, those in the precontemplation stage would not be yet ready for the demands required by a habit of health. Such folk would have no concept of a moral life and would most likely not be catechized into a life of faith. They would need formation first by the worshipping life of a Christian community. Such people would need to learn of Christ's love for them and would need to confess and receive forgiveness for their sins. Liturgical and communal action would provide the "consciousness" and support so that a person would be formed to even desire a life of virtue.

Contemplation

In this stage people acknowledge they want to change their behavior. They begin thinking about how they might initiate change and start making indefinite plans for action.[27] In Aquinas's paradigm, contemplation would represent the first movement of the will. A person begins deliberately concentrating upon a new habit they would like to cultivate. This disciplining of the will might begin through prayer; a person could initiate the directing the will to a new habit by offering it to God. Certainly they could recruit their passions around the habit and share their desire to make a change with friends.

If a person wants to begin a regular habit of running, for example, she could start by offering her desire to God in prayer. Through the discernment of prayer practices she could determine if running comprises a good new habit for her, and could begin envisioning her life with running in it. She could develop her own passion around running, supporting her

---

26. Ibid., 40–41, 89–90, 94. Prochaska, Norcross, and DiClemente advocate shifts within this stage by raising consciousness and becoming aware of defenses, often through helping relationships with others close to us or by "social liberation" groups. By liberation groups they mean self help groups like Alchoholic Anonymous.

27. Ibid., 42–43. Prochaska, Norcross, and Diclemente recommend that contemplators must arouse their emotions (get emotionally connected to the change they want to make) and perform a self-evaluation (taking stock of life and the needed change). Helping relationships provide invaluable support and truthfulness as a contemplator evaluates her behavior.

will through further prayer and discipline. She could also begin sharing her thoughts about a running practice with friends.

Preparation

People in the preparation stage make final adjustments to their behavior so that they are ready to begin something new. They might announce to friends and family that they are making a change.[28] They make a commitment to their coming habit, and begin changing their environment, gathering supplies, and creating a plan of action so that they can successfully execute their new behavior.

For practitioners of a new habit of health, preparation might represent the harnessing of the power of reason to the will to act virtuously. The reason acts as the person begins thinking about the performance of the new habit. Her reason moves her to buy new running shoes and a watch/heart rate monitor combo. With her reason she reads blogs and magazines on running, and finds a local running group she can join on Saturday mornings.

Action

Prochaska, Norcross, and DiClemente put action next. This stage describes the greatest overt changes in behavior and surroundings. People are committing time and energy to make the change in their life.[29] They are actually doing the new habit.

For Aquinas, a person must create enough potentiality through reason to develop a habit. By repeated cycles through contemplation and preparation (the will and reason), the person eventually builds up enough power to launch a new habit. The passive potential of the fresh habit then moves the appetitive power (will) toward action. In a Thomist sense, action only comes after a long build-up of the appetitive powers that creates a habit.

For our runner, she eventually builds up enough potential energy with her will and reason that on a Friday night she sets her alarm clock, puts out her running gear and an energy bar, and goes to sleep planning on getting up to run. When the alarm goes off the next morning, the

28. Ibid., 43.
29. Ibid., 44.

passive potential is great enough to get her up, out the door, and to the meeting site of the local running group. As she warms up, and then begins the first steps of her run, the appetitive power moves into the action. Her new habit has fully functioned for the first time.

Maintenance

In this stage people work to consolidate the gains attained during the action and other stages, and struggle to prevent lapses and relapse. Maintenance comprises a long, ongoing stage, which always retains the possibility of regression.[30] They must continue to internalize and act upon the lessons and growth from their journey through change.

For Thomas, maintenance could describe the life of virtue. Such a life requires ongoing vigilance so that habits don't diminish or corrupt. In order to sustain a habit of health a person must continue desiring to practice it, and maintain their same or higher level of intensity in their execution.

The runner, in other words, can't just desire to get up early one Saturday morning and run. For running to become a true habit, she must want to run regularly and consistently. She must set the alarm clock, put on her running gear, and get out to meet her running group at least weekly. In order to maintain the habit, she must maintain the intensity of her practice—which at first might be hard as she works to overcome years of not having such a habit. Through continuous maintenance over time, though, getting up early on Saturday morning becomes easier—it's just what she does, because she has become a runner. The habit, though perhaps difficult to launch and maintain in the beginning, becomes part of her nature.

Prochaska, Norcross, and DiClemente's model, while not perfect, does provide a clear, systematic way of understanding how a person might create healthy change in her life. When the psychologists' stages are combined with Aquinas's understanding of action through the will, reason, and habit, a helpful model emerges as to how someone can actually begin to practice a new habit of health. In this example, a person develops into a runner through cultivating a *habitus* by the repetitive movement of will and reason. This "dance" of the appetitive powers in

---

30. Ibid., 45–48. The authors assert that a person must accomplish certain tasks in each stage before moving on and can become stuck in a stage or regress backwards.

beginning and sustaining a healthy habit slowly shapes a person to become virtuous. In the next chapter we'll explore why we should devote ourselves to the cultivation of habits of health; in other words, what is health for in the Christian life?

8

What Is Health For? The Ends of Habits of Health

THUS FAR WE HAVE EXPLORED HOW AQUINAS ADAPTS ARISTOTELIAN habit and applies it in a virtuous practice of health. We have learned how the anthropology of habits supports agency in health, how our passions contribute to our health, and how we might actually cultivate habits of health. All of this exploration of habit and health leads to a *telos* in Aquinas's thought—an end toward which the practice of healthy habits can lead us. It is an end worth the effort of virtuous habits. It is the end of God welcoming us into deeper friendship and love, or beatitude.[1]

Below we'll first acknowledge the theological (faith, hope, and love) virtues, which enable Christians to pursue a moral life oriented to God. We'll then explore how the cardinal virtues (prudence, justice, courage, and temperance), when infused with the gifts of faith, hope, and love, enable us to cultivate health. Lastly we'll examine the role sickness plays in a Thomistic teleology. The practice of health as a part of the virtuous life means that habits of health can lead us deep into the heart of God—ultimately to a eudaimonistic life of happiness.

---

1. For Thomas, different lifestyles can purse different ways to the end of happiness in God. Aquinas, *ST* I-II 1–5. see also Wieland, "Happiness," 60. "[Aquinas] recognizes in principle the different ways in which this one end can be reached." However, this supernatural end can only be reached by those who accept the infused theological virtues of faith, hope, and love—or believers. For Aquinas pagans may indeed cultivate acquired virtues of prudence, temperance, courage, and justice, but they aren't oriented to the ultimate end of beatitude in God, and thus can be part of a divided self still immersed in vice. Aquinas, *ST* I-II 65.2. I'm also grateful for insights on the relationship between the infused acquired virtues, acquired virtues, and theological virtues from Overmyer, *The Wayfarer's Way*, 2010.

The Virtuous Life

The Theological Virtues

Habits of health participate in a community of moral virtues called the "acquired virtues," which develop through human dedication and effort, but are, for Christians, infused with the theological virtues of love, hope, and faith. The theological virtues come only as gifts from the Holy Spirit and enable humans to attain supernatural ends.[2] Growth in faith, hope, and love constitute the Christian life, and thus are foundational for understanding before we can speak of the practice of virtuous habits such as health.[3]

Thomas examines faith first, and articulates faith as a gift of God's grace that allows for a human being to assent with his mind, as directed by his will, to divine authority. Faith offers a conviction of the truth of the Christian faith, which retains both an inner consent, and an outer confession of what one believes.[4] For Thomas, faith allows Christians to accept as their fulfillment an end in the beatitude of God.[5]

Hope comes next for Aquinas as the theological virtue that is "grace-inspired confidence" that a believer receives from God.[6] For Thomas, hope empowers a believer so that she believes she will indeed reach the good of *eudiamonia*, or beatitude, in God. "Hope gives the believer a confident movement toward the future that enables him or her to overcome everything that restricts this movement to God."[7]

Out of all the theological virtues the third one, charity, comprises the bedrock in Thomas's schema. He writes that "there can be no true virtue without charity."[8] Charity mothers the virtues by bringing them to life as an expression of the intimacy we have with God.[9] In charity people

---

2. Aquinas, *ST* I-II 61.4. Thus the theological virtues are always infused by God's grace for Thomas.

3. Pope, "Overview of the Ethics of Thomas Aquinas," 37.

4. Ibid., 38.

5. Brown, "The Theological Virtue of Faith," 225.

6. Pope, "Overview of the Ethics of Thomas Aquinas," 38.

7. Ibid.

8. Aquinas, *ST* II-II 23.7. Pope, "Overview of the Ethics of Thomas Aquinas," 39. Faith offers belief in God and hope enables us to love God as the source of our happiness. However only charity forms us so that we love God as an end in himself. Kent, "Habits and Virtues," 122.

9. Considerable debate exists within Thomist studies as to whether the acquired

obtain the end for which they exist. Thomas considers love the "mother of all the virtues" because it conceives in them the desire of the ultimate end and charges them with life for that end.[10]

Thus, love dwells as the foundation of any of the acquired virtues. Charity makes the moral virtues into pathways for Christians to God.[11] Charity gives us the graced ability to cultivate friendship with God as our end. Consequently, charity enables us to love what God loves–our neighbor and ourselves. By having the right end (friendship/love of God) through charity we are empowered to live a virtuous life, which includes the ability to care for the health of ourselves and of others as an act of charity. Together all the theological virtues of faith, hope, and love permit us to accept our end in God, to overcome any impediments to that end, and to desire that end of friendship with God as what constitutes flourishing in life. With these virtues infused within us by grace, we can then begin to practice the moral life.[12]

The Acquired Virtues and Health

The four acquired virtues form a hinge upon which the moral life turns.[13] These virtues give each to the other mutual aid, working together in harmony to render a person "good."[14] These virtues of prudence, justice,

---

virtues can be obtained without the gift of charity or the infusion of the theological virtues. Scholars promulgate so-called public ethics in the acquired virtues that aren't infused. See Sheryl Overmyer, *Wayfarer's Way*, for a deep elaboration of the differences in Thomas of acquired virtues, acquired infused virtues, and theological virtues. I follow Dr. Amy Laura Hall's reading when she states that it would be cruelty to imagine that we could practice the acquired virtues without the first gift of love. Hall, "Christian Ethics."

10. Aquinas, *ST* II-II 23.8

11. Ibid., I-II 65.4 For pagans without charity, they may attempt to practice the acquired moral virtues, but the virtues cannot adhere to each other because they aren't united by and end in God.

12. This is to practice the moral life as Christians. We may begin to practice the moral life as pagans, but we could not end with friendship in God. For Aquinas, the virtuous life with God as an end is the more perfect way; for pagans the virtues always remain imperfect. Overmyer, *Wayfarer's Way*, 73, 76.

13. Wadell, *Primacy of Love*, 128. Cardinal comes from a Latin root which means "doorhinge."

14. Torrell, *Aquinas's Summa*, 46. "Insofar as any act is a virtue, it is also prudence, justice, temperance, and fortitude. In order for an act to be virtuous, we must be able to look at it and see each of these four qualities at work." Wadell, *Primacy of Love*, 129.

temperance, and fortitude guide virtuous human action, which includes health, and leads to the end of happiness—provided for first by the theological virtues.[15]

As a habit, the practice of health participates in all of the cardinal virtues, which affirms the unity of them. One practice might emphasize one virtue more than another, but a person's complete set of habits of health will function within all four of the acquired virtues. A person's habits of health lead her to be more prudent, just, courageous, and temperate. In order to argue that habits of health lead to a virtuous life throughout the cardinals, we'll again take up Gena's habit of running and examine it through each virtue, beginning with the virtue of prudence.

Prudence

Prudence perfects reason and enables the right judgment about things to be done.[16] Prudence supplies discernment and wisdom for our choices and enables a person to "see" things rightly so that we embody the good out of our deliberations.[17] It is the virtue of choice and decision.[18] Prudence grants artistry in the moral life so that decisions are not rote and mechanistic but rather part of the crafting of a good life.[19] Prudence guides the use of our minds and bodies so that we choose rightly what is good for our best health.[20]

Prudence guides Gena as she envisions what kind of training program would best suit her mind and body.[21] Rather than overtraining

---

Again, this unity in the virtues occurs only if they are of the kind infused with faith, hope, and love—especially love. Without love, the virtues literally fall apart. Overmyer, *The Wayfarer's Way*, 77.

15. Aquinas, *ST* I-II 61.2.

16. Ibid., I-II, 57.4, 71.1

17. Mattison, *Introducing Moral Theology*, 98. It is also considered an intellectual virtue without which moral virtue cannot exist; moral virtue consists of habits about good choosing. Prudence requires the rightness of appetites so that a person is rightly disposed with regard to their ends. Aquinas, *ST* I-II 57.4.

18. Torrell, *Aquinas's Summa*, 44.

19. Aquinas, *ST* I-II 57.5. Through the gift of God's love in charity we are able to love more completely as prudence guides us to overcome any hindrances of the passions.

20. Mattison, *Introducing Moral Theology*, 98. It is not merely knowing the good, but also embodying that good based upon deliberation.

21. Ibid., 101. Prudence, like any aquired virtue, is executed in mind and body.

due to an ambition to win, as many endurance runners are prone to do, Gena's deliberations through prudence guide her to a sensible program that allows for rest and offers a balance of speed work and long-distance. Through the practice of prudence Gena gains artistry in becoming a great athlete.[22] With the correct vision Gena chooses well how to train so that she runs prudently, resulting in less injuries and greater health. Such healthy acts trained by prudence help Gena, or any Christian, fit their habits into the whole of their life, oriented to a happy end.

Justice

Aquinas defines justice as *"suum cuique,"* which means to render to each her due according to *jus*, or what is right or proper.[23] It describes doing what needs to be done in the way it needs to be done.[24] Right, or *jus*, exists when one creature's relationship to another allows for the satisfaction of their natural needs. Injustice would include thinking ill of another person without sufficient reason and backbiting, for example. The virtue of justice affirms Aristotle's maxim that we are social animals and that a good life consists of flourishing with others. Our own happiness remains inextricable from the common good of others.[25] Practices of health uphold justice when the physical/emotional/spiritual needs of the most vulnerable in our midst are addressed and cared for.[26]

Gena's individual practice of running doesn't readily seem to connect to justice. However, as a Christian Gena realizes that her own happiness, which she derives from running, remains inextricable from the common good of others around her.[27] Perhaps out of her love for running

22. Aquinas, *ST* I-II 57.5. Through prudence one gains artistry in the moral life so that decisions aren't rote and mechanistic but rather part of the crafting of a good life.

23. Ibid., I-II 136. The virtue of justice involves rendering to each person what is owed her voluntarily and constantly. Aquinas, *ST* I-II 58.1. Justice entails the sub-virtues of honesty, generosity, loyalty, and promise-keeping.

24. Ibid., I-II 61.4

25. Mattison, *Introducing Moral Theology*, 139–40.

26. For example, the fact that many of America's inner cities are food and activity deserts, in which people have little access to fresh foods or outdoor physical activity, comprises an injustice. Justice is rendered when the wealthy (taxpayers, community leaders, churches) work to establish grocery stores of healthy abundance in underserved communities and safe play areas for children without access to green space. Justice means that hungry bellies are filled with good things and energetic children have places to play.

27. Mattison, *Introducing Moral Theology*, 139–40.

she decides to volunteer with Girls on the Run, a national organization to promote habits of running in young girls in order to boost self-esteem, confidence, and health.[28] Her habit of health, then, contributes to and supports the development of good habits in the vulnerable population of pre-teen girls—and justice is cultivated.

In addition, Gena's own participation in her church and its worship ensures that she is rendering to God what is due God—doxology.[29] Such a practice of justice prevents Gena from pride in her own athletic accomplishments. Justice supports Gena to an end of deeper relationship with God, and of a loving relationship with her neighbor.

Temperance

Temperance is the most inherently bodily virtue, and most directly relatable to habits of health. Temperance describes the mean between vices of concupiscence and frigidity and is directed to the emotions and tempers them so that they are not either too much, making us impetuous, or too little, rendering us apathetic.[30] Aquinas, following Aristotle, affirms that temperance most often guides the pleasures of food, drink, and sex—though it also includes anything we long for or desire.[31] A temperate person desires and enjoys food, drink, sex and other pleasures in the mean—not too little and not too much.[32] Health, obviously, comes when people practice the mean so that they don't become overweight or underweight, frigid or licentious.

Temperance is also bodily, and thus concerns health, because of the centrality of the passions within this virtue. Temperance balances our emotions and enables us to act fittingly.[33] As we inhabit bodies filled with longings and hungers, temperance trains us as to how best direct their

28. See www.girlsontherun.org.

29. Pope, "Overview of the Ethics of Thomas Aquinas," 42.

30. Wadell, *Primacy of Love*, 133.

31. Ibid., 76. Temperance includes both the well-ordered desire for pleasures, and the actual partaking of them. The virtue of temperance acknowledges that we are creatures of incredible drives and passions, and seeks to refine, direct, and discipline those passions to serve virtue.

32. Ibid., 78. The vice of intemperance is most often a matter of excessive desire for pleasures, but can also be an issue of too little desire. An intemperate person, for example, might eat too little such that her health and life are put at risk.

33. Ibid., 134–35. Wadell describes how temperance erodes the power of shameful emotional forces and trains us toward beauty—which represents proper measure and proportion in our actions.

energies. In addition temperance teaches us to not only to act well, but also to have the right desires in acting well. "The temperate person not only does the right thing for the right reason but also desires to do it from her heart."[34]

The virtue of temperance teaches that Gena shouldn't run out of obligation or guilt, even if the exercise still accomplishes her goal of improved health and fitness. Instead, temperance trains Gena to exercise out of motivations of pleasure and enjoyment. She runs (in the mean—not excessively to injury, or insufficiently so she derives no benefit) because she delights in the running. The virtue of temperance means Gena practices a habit of health because it ultimately brings her joy, and that joy connects to the ultimate joy experienced in a life lived toward God.

Courage

Courage names the habit that enables us to face difficulties well and to "readily endure all for the sake of what is loved."[35] Fortitude, or courage, grants emotional stability to every other virtue as it strengthens us to be steadfast and not turn away from what is right.[36] Courage helps us to stand our ground amidst dangers and persevere in times of hardship for what we love and don't want to lose. Fortitude helps us to continue even when it is not possible to see the end of our work—or our lives.[37]

In Gena's case, she might call upon courage during a marathon race in which she is filled with fear and doubt about being able to finish. At mile nineteen when she "hits the wall" and feels she can no longer go on, Gena summons fortitude and endures through the remaining seven

---

34. Mattison, *Introducing Moral Theology*, 88. Mattison cites Aquinas, *ST* I-II 24.3 for this statement.

35. Aquinas, *ST* II-II 23.4. Mattison, *Introducing Moral Theology*, 180.

36. Pope, "Overview of the Ethics of Thomas Aquinas," 43. The Christian martyr exemplifies courage through her willingness to offer her life for the witness to God's kingdom, but courage is found also in everyday, quotidian experiences in life as well. Fortitude strengthens us from fear of danger and hardship to what reason requires. It enables us to move forward to the good in the midst of danger and death.

37. Aquinas *ST* I-II 61.2. Fortitude functions in unity with all the other cardinal virtues; it grants the emotional stability to exercise every other virtue. A courageous person needs prudence in order to determine how to act well, to know which good is more or less important. Without justice, bravery could be truly cruel. Without temperance, a person could be inordinately attracted to sensible pleasures and then be incapable of confronting difficulties and dangers as well. Pope, "Overview of the Ethics of Thomas Aquinas," 43, 184.

miles with sore feet and aching muscles.³⁸ This athletic practice of fortitude may seem individualistic, yet such a summoning of courage during a race easily translates into challenges in life. Out of her experience of perseverance in the contest, Gena is formed so that she can more readily endure through the terminal illness of a beloved, or through the loss of a job. Courage in the practice of habits of health literally renders us more fit so that we can persevere through suffering in life. Bravery on behalf of our own health translates into a greater ability to be brave for the sake of faithfulness to the Gospel. By refusing to live in fear, whether on a race course or in an emergency room, Christians endure with perseverance for the sake of the ultimate end.

In summation, then, the practice of habits of health renders us more prudent, just, temperate, and courageous. As inseparable as the cardinal virtues are from each other, so too is the habit of health interwoven with the practice of all of them. Health represents a legitimate proximate end, but must be ordered properly to the ultimate end. In answering the question "what are habits of health for" the response might be, such healthy habits comprise a holistic (body, mind, and spirit) way to live more deeply into the virtuous life—a life made possible by the graced gifts of faith, hope, and love—so that our lives orient to beatitude. This virtuous life assists us on our journey as Christians into greater love of God.

Teleology and Sickness

Within this teleology, then, we orient our health to the glory of God. Even those who are sick or disabled cultivate whatever health they may and direct that strength for life also to God. Yet a question still remains: if health has such a vital role in the virtuous life, what role then does sickness play? Is disease purely vice? Does it serve any end?

In response, certainly sickness represents an affront to human life; it is in no way a good. It prevents us from living into the fullness of life we desire by hindering us with injury, pain, or disability.³⁹ Sickness represents an envoy of a powerful enemy—death. Disease and its minions threaten us with the power of chaos, disorder, and danger.

---

38. "Hitting the wall" is a phrase used by distance runners to describe a state of complete exhaustion and depletion of energy (glycogen) resources. For marathoners miles 18–20 are usually when they feel they can no longer go on . . . yet must still summon the energy to go seven more miles.

39. Barth, *Doctrine of Creation*, 357.

However, those who undergo the brutal attacks of sickness must not be judged as themselves vicious. Christ himself guards against such thinking when he clarifies that a young man wasn't sick out of his sinfulness (John 9). While the schema of habits of health definitely affirms that we have responsibility for our health, it also allows that each of us is born differently, some with greater health than others.[40] Since the etiology of disease for many conditions remains shrouded in mystery and each of our individual constitutions interacts differently in our environment, judgment must be withheld from the sick.

Could sickness, even as a forerunner of death, possibly then serve a role in the virtuous life? While Aquinas doesn't specifically elaborate on any benefits from sickness in the *Treatise on Habit*, Pope John Paul II in his apostolic letter *Salvifici Doloris*, does. The Holy Father reads Colossians 1:24—"I rejoice in my sufferings for your sake"—as an *urtext* for the salvific meaning of suffering in union with Christ. The Pope writes of a sick person that, "Faith in sharing the suffering of Christ brings with it the interior certainty that in the spiritual dimensions of the work of Redemption he is serving, like Christ, the salvation of his brothers and sisters. Therefore he is carrying out an irreplaceable service."[41] Through a person's experience of suffering in sickness, she makes present the power of the Redemption, united to the redemptive suffering of Christ. She becomes a witness to the power of good and the victory of that salvific power through her virtuous courage and endurance.[42] Such a witness does not burden a sick person with something else to have to do, but rather the work of testimony overcomes the sense of the uselessness of suffering. By completing "what is lacking in Christ's afflictions" (Col 1:24) the sick person shines forth to others the true joy of Christ's triumph over the powers of death and darkness that sicknesses represent.

The sufferer can discover then a new vocation and character out of the experience of sickness. She nurtures her newly acquired life's work through the use of habits that sustain virtues. In cultivating courage for her nascent work of witness, she experiences hope in God that the suffering will not better her, and will not deprive her of her dignity as a human being.[43] She lives into a deeper peace and spiritual joy than she knew

---

40. Aquinas, *ST* I-II 51.1.

41. John Paul II, *Salvifici Doloris* under the section, "The Gospel of Suffering."

42. Ibid.

43. Ibid., under "Sharers in the Suffering of Christ."

before her illness and is able to love others more compassionately.[44] Her way out of the darkness of suffering through illness leads into a lit path filled with loving service to others.[45] The sick person can receive true holiness as a gift out of the sickness. While sickness itself remains an evil, a person can live into a deeper, richer, more virtuous life out of such an evil. God can use even the opposite of health to bring about greater health and a profoundly virtuous life. This virtuous life offers the possibility of the practice of health even in sickness, and directs the practitioner to an end of deep life-giving happiness, even with an illness that portends death.

Conclusion

In the end, Aquinas's understanding of the role of virtue in health directs all of us, whether sick or well or in-between, to an end of deeper joy and happiness.[46] Aquinas's model of healthy habits offers to us a sacred orientation directed ultimately into the heart of God. The love of God then becomes the end (*telos*) of health practices, so that health itself never becomes the *summum bonum*, but the result of a life focused on the right end.

Practices of habits of health shape us so that not only do we become healthier in our bodies and souls, but we also become more virtuous. Through cultivating health we find ourselves becoming more prudent, more just, more courageous, and more temperate. Health becomes part of our character.

In the next chapters we will examine two specific Christian communities who have been cultivating more virtuous, healthy lives. Neither of them intentionally appropriated Aquinas's understanding of habit, but both communities (in different ways) demonstrate what it might look like for Christians to care for their health as though their lives depended upon it. It is to their witness that we now turn.

44. Barth, *Doctrine of Creation*, 374. Barth states that in sickness we are drawn by God and by our own will for life into a deeper joy, delight, and happiness.

45. This in many ways describes the way of the mystic, demonstrated in the work of Spanish Carmelite John of the Cross (sixteenth century) and Hadewijch (Dutch Beguine, early to mid 1200s).

46. Torrell, *Aquinas's Summa*, 40. Torrell offers the insight that Thomas's orientation is to the positive. Though he recognizes sin, Thomas upholds the power of God's grace. This is a marked contrast to the impulses undergirding much of the Christian "self-improvement" dieting books, which strongly emphasize sinfulness in eating. Griffiths, *Born Again Bodies*, 207.

PART TWO

Habits of Health in Christian Community

9

Clergy Health Initiative

An Introduction to the Study of Ecclesial Communities

AMERICAN CLERGY HAVE BEEN SHOWN TO STRUGGLE MORE THAN THE general population with chronic health issues. Studies indicate that clergy strain under enormous levels of stress from unrealistic time demands, emotional exhaustion, low work satisfaction, lack of family time and privacy, and high expectations from parishoners, just to name a few.[1] Due to these pressures and often inadequate social support systems for themselves (strong, trustworthy friendships, etc.) clergy can often experience depression and acute anxiety.[2] Despite in general having high levels of spiritual wellbeing and the use of a wide array of spiritual resources (prayer, worship, etc.), the demanding nature of their vocation compromises the robust spiritual health religious professionals usually cultivate.[3]

---

1. Rowatt, "Stress and Satisfaction in Ministry Families," 523–43. Rowatt categorized four main areas of stress: 1. Vocational stressors (inadequate pay, low work satisfaction, unrealistic time demands, relocation) 2. Intrapersonal stressors (emotional exhaustion, burnout, low personal satisfaction, sense of personal failure) 3. Family stressors (low family satisfaction, lack of family time, lack of privacy) 4. Social stressors (high expectations regarding behavior, criticism, intrusiveness, and lack of social support). See also Lee and Iverson-Gilbert. "Demand, Support, and Perception," 249–57. These researchers classify clergy stress into personal criticism, boundary ambiguity, presumptive expectations, and family criticism. They view these causes of stress as lowering pastoral wellbeing and leading to greater pastor burn-out. See also Proeschold-Bell et al., "Theoretical Model of the Holistic Health of United Methodist Clergy."

2. Turton and Francis, "Relationship between Attitude toward Prayer," 61–74. This study noted that 30 percent of clergy had experienced depression, and 21 percent acute anxiety since ordination.

3. Meisenhelder and Chandler, "Frequency of Prayer," 323–29. This study indicated

PART TWO—Habits of Health in Christian Community

For example, among United Methodist clergy in North Carolina, more suffer from obesity (79 percent), diabetes, arthritis, asthma, and high blood pressure than the general population.[4] If any population stands to benefit from a Thomist-based practice of habits of health, it would be religious professionals such as clergy—whose very work puts their health at greater risk.

Since clergy serve as leaders in their respective Christian communities and contend not only with cultural but also vocational obstacles to health, it makes sense that if they can cultivate habits of health that promote greater flourishing, then most other Christians can, too—plus they serve a vital modeling role for their faith communities. In order to reflect more deeply on how habits of health might practically influence Christians' experience of wellbeing, I investigated two communities that have instituted programs to enhance the health of their members. The Clergy Health Initiative (CHI), which focuses upon United Methodist clergy in North Carolina, and the Community Care ministry within the evangelical missionary organization Word Made Flesh (WMF); WMF will be analyzed in the next chapter. Both programs, though, nurtured practices among their members that resulted in greater holistic health and more virtuous lives.

In order to describe these programs and the changes they wrought in people's lives, I'll begin this chapter by offering an introduction to Clergy Health Initiative (CHI). I'll then briefly describe my methods of research, and analyze the results of my interviews with CHI participants, presenting their barriers to health, theology of the body, new habits that emerged out of CHI, and a discussion of the data. (Larger conclusions about the church and its need to cultivate habits of health that came out of this study will be discussed in the concluding chapter.)

Though not intentionally Thomist in their philosophy of health, these faith groups reveal through their innovative programs how habits of health bring transformation and greater love of God, neighbor, and self into real people's lives. The two programs embody Thomas's insights that good habits make us more fully into who we are created to be and

---

that higher frequency of prayer correlates to better levels of mental health in clergy. (Admittedly, some of these studies which I'm citing constitute part of the problem of science's analysis of religion.)

4. www.divinity.duke.edu/initiatives-centers/clergy-health-initiative-ongoing research, and www.divinity.duke.edu/initiatives-centers/clergy-health-initiative/learning under "What We are Learning."

guide us into God's graced promises for our lives.[5] The clergy of CHI and the missionaries of WMF serve as exemplars of Aquinas's understanding of habituation. Through their practices of health they do indeed become more virtuous, happy people. The interviewees became more patient, kinder to their families, and more vital in their ministries—all because they started exercising, or eating better, or taking a regular personal retreat. Thomas's theology represents the hermeneutical key that unlocks why such transformations happened from changes in daily habits. The religious leaders admit themselves that they aren't sufficiently and fully habituated into health, and so Thomas's model serves as further catechesis for those on the journey toward lives of flourishing--while at the same time affirming the ethical renovations they have made as individuals and as communities.

Introduction to Clergy Health Initiative

The Clergy Health Initiative (CHI) represents a $12 million, seven year program designed to improve the health and wellbeing of over 1600 United Methodist clergy serving in North Carolina; it represents a partnership between Duke Divinity School, the Duke Endowment, the Western North Carolina and North Carolina Conferences of the United Methodist Church and is part of Leadership Education at Duke Divinity School.[6] The program began by researchers conducting eleven clergy focus groups (88 people) and fielded a survey that 95% of clergy in NC completed (1,726 people). Based upon the sobering results of this fieldwork CHI launched a pilot program with 81 pastors in the Goldsboro district of the North Carolina conference and the Northeast district (Reidsville area) of the Western North Carolina conference.[7] With a focus upon agency, the 12 month program provided for the participants the following resources: lab tests, two 45 minute physical exams by a doctor with follow-up, a health coach, up to $1,190 in money for services to support health (gym membership, fitness equipment, counseling, etc.), support for the formation of Wesleyan bands (small groups), and access to health education.[8]

---

5. Aquinas, *ST* I-II 49.2. Wadell, *Primacy of Love*, 136.
6. Clergy Health Initiative, "Ongoing Research."
7. Ibid.
8. Ibid.

PART TWO—Habits of Health in Christian Community

The experiences of those clergy who participated in the now-completed pilot program serve as the basis for my research.[9]

Methodology

I chose to collect data through personal interviews with clergy participants in CHI's pilot program—all of whom had completed the program by the time of the interview.[10] In total I had ten interviews with four clergy from the Goldsboro district and six from the Northeastern district (Reidsville area); gender distribution was six males and four females.[11] Interview questions consisted of nine structured questions and focused upon the clergyperson's theology of the body/health, hindrances to his/her care of her health, a Wesleyan and Thomist understanding of healthcare, and reflections upon their experience in the Clergy Health Initiative's pilot program.[12]

Data analysis began after all interviews were completed and was the same process for CHI and Word Made Flesh (WMF). I sought regularities in the data and derived coding categories from the data rather than from any predetermined hypothesis.[13] I developed themes out of patterns and repetitions in the data, and grouped those themes into larger domains to

---

9. Based upon the insights received from the pilot program, CHI launched Spirited Life in January 2011, a multi-year health/wellness/and behavioral health program offered to all United Methodist clergy in North Carolina, providing resources for spiritual renewal, stress management, healthy/mindful eating, coaching/support, and behavioral health within a framework of Wesleyan theology and spirituality. See http://spiritedlife.org.

10. The participants from both districts were recruited via email from a CHI staff person; the clergy had to voluntarily contact me from that email. Out of the recruitment email I received twelve responses, and coordinated via email with the clergy in order to set up a meeting time and place (usually the pastor's church).

11. Nine of the clergy were elders (ordained with a Master of Divinity degree) and one was a local pastor (completed a course of study program). I conducted the interviews during January 3–5, 2011, with the interviews organized by area.

12. The questions remained the same throughout the ten interviews. After conducting the ten interviews themes raised by the participants had reached the point of redundancy, or saturation, so I decided not to conduct further phone interviews with the two clergy unable to meet in person during the week I was in North Carolina. The interviews lasted for 60–90 minutes and the Duke University Institutional Review Board approved the study. All interviews were audiotaped and verbatim notes were also taken during the interview.

13. Charmaz, "Grounded Theory," 335–52. Proeschold-Bell et al., "Theoretical Model of the Holistic Health of United Methodist Clergy," under Methods.

help organize and make sense of the data.¹⁴ An analysis of the data from both programs follows below.

Hindrances to Healthcare for Clergy

I asked questions about barriers clergy experienced in cultivating good health in order to develop greater understanding of all the health challenges clergy face. The number and severity of barriers to good health in clergy's lives illuminates why so many struggle with chronic disease.

No Catechesis in Health from Church during Childhood

To a person, those clergy who were raised in the United Methodist Church received no formation around topics of health and the body. As one pastor put it, "it was formation by lack of formation." A common refrain from the pastors was stated by one whose father was a United Methodist clergy, "I can't remember anything from the church about health." By the church's negligence in teaching on the body, these pastors could have imbibed as children that their health and bodies weren't significant or deserving of attention.¹⁵ This lack of teaching on health during their formative years may have influenced clergy as adults to value other commitments more than their healthcare.

Time Management and Constant Availability

Many pastors mentioned the challenge of managing their time due to the enormous amount of responsibilities they juggle. Clergy view themselves as overloaded with work and live with a pervasive sense of never getting everything done, often trading off sleep, exercise, and a good diet in order

---

14. I identified four domains in the CHI research: hindrances to care of health for clergy, including theological barriers, theology of the body, including Scripture, the potential of Aquinas's theology for the health of clergy, and new habits of health out of CHI participation. The domains for each program form the basis of my analysis, which follows next.

15. The only positive mention of health formation in the church came from a pastor who experienced a Presbyterian summer church camp that emphasized good nutrition. A couple of pastors raised in the Baptist tradition stated that their formation around the body emphasized the sinfulness of drug and alcohol use, as well as the dangers of being overweight; this catechesis taught that the body constituted a site of peril.

PART TWO—Habits of Health in Christian Community

to complete tasks, lead meetings, or prepare sermons. One clergyperson described the demands and pressures of the profession in this way:

> The mindset of pastors is to take care of people all the time. Our work is never finished so we end up denying self. I don't know if it is the work that does it to us or if we get into the work because we have it in us—where if we don't work we feel guilty. The list of duties in the *Discipline* is crazy; there is no way to do it all. . . .Within us and according to the churches' demands of us is a heavy weight for the spiritual wellbeing of people. There is a real impetus to be active in people's lives.

The impetus to be involved in people's lives, a pressure which comes for pastors both internally and externally from their congregations, results in pastors feeling that they must be constantly available to serve their people. Many mentioned feeling that they were on a twenty-four hour/seven days a week work schedule because of their availability to parishoners.

> There is a sense of a 24/7 mentality of clergy. We cultivate the idea in ourselves, and we allow others to cultivate it in us, that we are—to quote Will Willimon—quivering masses of availability. There is something in us to be caring and nurturing and looking out for others. When we become focused on that, it leads detrimentally to not taking care of ourselves.

The interviewees were very aware of the pressures of their vocation and of their availability to people, yet also seemed (as the clergyperson quoted above) to be cognizant of how damaging such pressures are to their life and wellbeing. For most, though, they required CHI to support them in order to make actual changes in their management of time and presence to their parishoners. As Aquinas's understanding of the action of habit demonstrates, simply being aware of one's time pressures and constant availability isn't enough to evoke changes in habit.

"Savior Complex" and "Martyrdom"

Many clergy could identify with the pastor quoted above who described an internal impetus to be caring and nurturing, giving completely of oneself to others. The male clergy often described this trait as a "Savior complex" in which they must be a "superpastor" and try and be like Jesus. An interviewee described it this way:

> I do desire to be excellent at my work and I take my job seriously. Pastors stand in for Lord Jesus. When Jesus was asked to minister to someone he didn't say "I need to work out"... Jesus was always there for people, so we need to be there for people. A lot of this rests inside of me—my own desire to please and be like Jesus.

Another male clergyperson identified the pride and hubris that comes along with the "Savior complex;" clergy want their parishoners to notice how hard they are working and what sacrifices they are making to do excellent work. He described the savior complex this way:

> (Pastors think) if I take time for me I'm taking time away from the church. Pride is the issue here. (Pastors want the congregation to) Look at me—I've stayed at the hospital all night long. There is the idea that somehow we are to be superpastors, which is a prideful thing and a generational thing. It goes by osmosis from older pastors to younger—we must become this... We don't go home, we eat whatever people give us. All of that keeps pastors from good health.

Female clergy, in describing similar desires to serve and do outstanding work used the word "martyrdom" instead of "savior complex." Instead of pride, they described feeling guilt if they didn't do everything possible in a day to nurture their parishoners. They question, "Did I do enough? Should I have made that phone call?" They feel they have to give so much that they inevitably deplete themselves, even though they recognize that such exhaustion isn't faithful either. One clergywoman said:

> There is a sense that we are supposed to martyr ourselves, a sense that a true pastor is worn out and broken down. There is an idea of martyrdom so that if you aren't doing that then you aren't giving your all. Yet in scripture Jesus was not always available—he did go aside to pray...

Aside from clergywomen's internal pressures, the congregation can also perpetuate the sense of martyrdom. One clergywoman's summer intern (a seminary student from Duke Divinity School) was told by a parishoner that "she (meaning the female pastor) is called to die for us." Obviously, overt affirmations of martyrdom and clergy's own internal pressures to live sacrificially coalesce to form highly detrimental influences to health, severely inhibiting any efforts to cultivate good habits.

PART TWO—Habits of Health in Christian Community

People Pleasers

Closely connected to both the difficulties with time management and the savior/martyrdom complex are many clergypersons' desires to please their parishoners and be liked/affirmed by those they serve. Several clergy mentioned wanting to be liked by their congregations and wanting to please. One clergyperson in a rural area stated that he was worried about what people would think if he took time to work out because he serves a church culture in which most people don't exercise—he didn't want to do anything that would upset them or cause them to think he wasn't working hard enough. Another stated:

> We pastors need to be seen and loved and appreciated. In the end it is vaporous and insipid. In the end the *telos* is you.

This pastor made the theological connection that the desire to please others really comes out a misplaced need for a greater self, rather than a focus on God. Such desires to please others by sacrificing one's health are, quite ironically, much more selfish than the desire to care for one's health. As the clergyperson indicated, a *telos* of oneself prevents a person from ever reaching more substantive ends—namely, as Aquinas teaches, a *telos* of friendship with God.

The United Methodist Appointment System[16]

Several pastors mentioned the United Methodist system of appointment as contributing to poor health in a myriad of different ways. One felt that the guaranteed appointment system, in which ordained elders are assured a post at a church and from which they cannot easily be fired, can promote spiritual laziness and a lackadaisical attitude toward health disciplines.[17] Another felt that the appointment system often places young, promising pastors in small rural, dysfunctional charges where no opportunities for relationships with people their age exist—and these churches

---

16. In the United Methodist Church, which is organized by conferences, bishops and district superintendents (called the Cabinet of the conference), the Cabinet in consultation with churches and pastors, decide where pastors will serve. In the UMC's itinerant system clergy are moved frequently, often every three to seven years.

17. This system of guaranteed appointment was under review by the last General Conference (2012), the overarching legislative body of the United Methodist church. The Conference decided to eliminate guaranteed appointment for elders, but this decision is under review.

constrain the pastor to maintain archane, dying programs. Such grim appointments deaden a person's passion for ministry and compromise their health in a few years. One pastor with children describes her situation this way:

> When I think about the reality of what God wants for me, it doesn't look like a full time pastorate by myself in a rural church. My appointment doesn't match any reality of self-care and abundant life . . . if I could job share that would make this doable. Our paradigm isn't set up for clergy to be healthy. I agree with Aquinas but I feel stuck. I am not going to be able to meet expectations and take care of myself the way God intends.

Her truthful lament names the complex challenges of the appointment system within the United Methodist Church that compromise clergy's ability to live into flourishing. Even if pastors were able to overcome individual hindrances to health, they still face prospects of serving churches and living in communities entirely ill-suited to their gifts and graces.

Theological Hindrances

Clergy articulated a couple of theological hindrances that they felt prevented them from vibrant lives of health. Several mentioned a pervasive Cartesian dualism, which separates the mind from the body and elevates the mind/spirit/soul as higher and more deserving of care than the body. Rural clergy, especially in revivalist churches, articulated that in their congregations the "health of the spirit is all that matters" and that parishoners often think, "I am a soul and just live in the body" such that the body becomes a devalued container. In commenting on dualism in the church, a clergyperson stated:

> The biggest heresy for clergy is that our primary responsibility is to take care of people's minds . . . Christ and his ministry was much more holistic.

Interviewees also mentioned the heresy of Gnosticism as pervasive within the church. While no one elaborated on the specifics of this early church heresy, several (particularly women) invoked it to describe many Christians' desire to be "freed from bodies" or to "escape from the body." A clergywoman described the practice of Gnosticism in the church as the "sense that we should abuse the body by not taking care of it—a heretical party in the church." Gnosticism leads to the denigration of the body and the denial of the body as good. Clergy, while aware of these heresies (dualism/Gnosticism), perceived them as residing within the Methodist church culture or within their own parishes; no one articulated that he/she felt these heresies influenced their own attitudes toward their bodies.

However, the ways in which several of the clergy treated their bodies before the CHI intervention suggests that such theological hindrances might also be deeply embedded within clergy themselves. Such damaging theology, combined with all the other hindrances mentioned by clergy, makes for a particularly poisonous brew for clergy health.[18] These barriers to good health must be overcome in order for clergy to live flourishing lives; all of the clergy interviewed required the intervention of CHI in order to evoke change—the hindrances were too strong and many and the wills were not hardy enough to instigate new habits without an "outside mover."

Aquinas's theology certainly understands that changes in habits remain difficult and hindrances to virtue are legion; his account of the action of the will acknowledges that new habits require immense stamina. A Thomist account of habits of health recognizes that hindrances such as time management and a "martyr complex" must be openly known in order to be dealt with and eventually overcome.

Clergy's Theology of the Body

Despite all of the hindrances described above, clergy articulated a theological anthropology that affirmed embodiment as good. When asked about their theological understanding of the body and about any scriptures that guided their understanding of the care of health, several themes emerged from these United Methodist pastors. Common resonances within their theology comes as no surprise, given that seven out of the ten interviewees attended Duke Divinity School for their theological training.[19]

---

18. Other hindrances which were mentioned by only one or two clergy members include: the consumer economy in the church, cost of health insurance (since full elders receive health insurance this wasn't a personal financial concern, but a concern for the financial loss to the church from high medical claims), and the lack of access to fresh, organic food for rural clergy.

19. Out of the other three clergy, one attended Candler School of Theology at Emory University, one attended Southeastern Theological Seminary (Baptist), and

Called to Be Good Stewards

Over and over again the clergy described a notion of "stewardship of the body." By this they meant that as Christians we are called—we have a "spiritual imperative"—to care for our bodies. Pastors affirmed our bodies as "magnificent gifts from God" and indicated that faithfulness requires that we tend to them.

Called to Be Good Shepherds

Another common theological refrain was the vocation of shepherd. By this metaphor clergy were both referring to themselves as leaders of their congregations and indicating the imperative to be good role models for their people. They felt they couldn't be "good shepherds to the sheep" if they weren't living healthy lives. One interviewee stated:

> Anything that we proclaim and profess we need to model for our congregation. If we preach about prayer and devotional life (there is a problem) if they (the congregation) know we don't do this. It's the same thing for observing Sabbath, for rest and renewal...the same thing applies to healthy habits. Modeling goes a long way to forming a congregation—more than the words we speak.

Another pastor described how he was a better shepherd after the CHI participation:

> I am a shepherd modeling for the sheep; I model for the people. I encourage people to jog or walk on the street. My forty-pound weight loss is significant . . . people see the health and the spirit and the joy.

Clergy genuinely want to be exemplars of health for their people and that desire has solidly rooted foundations in their theological understanding of the pastor's role as shepherd.

---

one attended Asbury. The predominance of Duke educations comes as no surprise, given that it is located in Durham, NC—within driving distance of all of these clergy's parishes.

PART TWO—Habits of Health in Christian Community

God Created All Things Good

More than any other scripture, pastors cited the creation narrative of Genesis as affirming the goodness of the body. A pastor remarked that since God used the same raw materials of creation to make humankind, and all of that materiality is deemed good, then it also follows that human bodies are good. The God who cares about physical creation also cares about physical bodies and is concerned for their wellbeing. Health represents an essential part of creation. Within this scriptural account pastors also cited *imago dei*, or being made in the image of God, as a reason for tending to the body.

> God created us in his image and likeness. I don't see the body as an enemy or problem; It is proper and responsible to take care of it. It's very Wesleyan to attend to physical matters ... Creation is good. The body is a good thing.

The Body Is a Temple

Besides creation, the other most common scripture motif referred to the body as a temple of the Holy Spirit. Citing Paul (though none of the pastors indicated a specific text) the clergy repeatedly affirmed that the body is sacred and thus well-deserving of care. The interviewees strongly thought that Pauline theology articulates the importance of the body, not only as a residence of the Holy Spirit but also for athletic training that parallels spiritual disciplines (citing texts like running the race, training the body into submission, etc.). One clergywoman described her understanding of Pauline texts this way:

> Paul says the body is the temple of the Lord. I believe that the Holy Spirit resides in us. We are the place where God abides. I believe in taking care of myself and not abusing that privilege, so I eat correctly and drink the right thing.

Clergy overwhelmingly stated that the Bible supports tending to the body and interpreted Pauline texts as teaching that health is Godly.[20]

---

20. Another theme mentioned by two interviewees was the significance of the resurrection for the affirmation of the body; since Christ was inherently physical in the resurrection, such embodiment teaches that we too will always have our bodies. Other Scriptures cited only once include Ps 40, Deut 6:1–4, and Jer 29:11.

John Wesley's Practice of Holism

One of my questions began by offering background into John Wesley's theological and practical commitments to health and then asked how the Wesleyan heritage might help them care for their own wellbeing and that of their congregations.[21] Though most of the pastors were aware of Wesley's manual of self-help remedies, *Primitive Physic*, they weren't educated in the depth of his personal and theological dedication to holism.[22] Based mainly upon the information I shared through the preface to my Wesley question the clergy felt that Wesley was wisely prescient on matters of diet and exercise and that the founder's emphasis on personal and communal health inspired and encouraged them to continue in health practices. The interviewees felt that Wesley integrated theology with real human life through a holistic understanding of salvation, and lamented the loss of such Wesleyan theology in many United Methodist Churches today. On the possibility of teaching her congregation about John Wesley's affirmation of the significance of health for the Christian life a pastor said:

> People would want to hear me offer that John Wesley believed in this (holistic health) . . . People would find this (Wesley's theology/practice of health) liberating. We need permission to care for our bodies—that it is okay and not "unspiritual" to care for ourselves . . . For my own self it is inspirational. I knew that he (Wesley) was brilliant, but also he was so ahead of his time in caring for the poor and in finding ways to care for the body . . . We are about the whole body and whole lives—we are not just to deal with baptizing, marrying, and burying. There is a problem that everything (to do with health) has been outsourced . . . (Wesley's teachings) can help people to address issues and get help. This is a good thing.

Another pastor stated that Wesley would most likely demand for pastors to take care of themselves while another remarked that Wesleyan acts of piety would include not only prayer and conferencing but also diet and exercise. In summation, the interviewees practically rejoiced to learn of a Wesleyan heritage of healthcare and felt renewed in their own efforts at healthcare through learning about it.

---

21. See also my article on Wesley's commitment to integrated health. Melanie Dobson Hughes, "Holistic Way," 237–52.

22. See Maddox, "John Wesley on Holistic Health and Healing," 4–33.

PART TWO—Habits of Health in Christian Community

Thomas Aquinas's Theology of Habit

Like I did with the Wesley question, I provided a brief sketch in the interview of Thomas Aquinas's theology of health; though all of the interviewees were familiar with Aquinas, none of them were aware of any Thomist emphasis on health. With unanimity the pastors supported Aquinas's conception of habit as nurturing practices of health. They felt such theology was "right on target" and that habit was key for lives of wellbeing. One pastor felt that habit affirms the sense of health as a lifestyle for those created in the image of God in which spiritual, mental, and emotional health all play a role. Another remarked:

> The word habitual is important. It (health) does become habitual. If I don't exercise and eat properly it is like a week of missing worship . . . Habitually exercising, eating properly and seeing a physician are good habits. These are not for narcissism—again it comes to mind that most of society, when they think of eating healthy and exercising it is for narcissistic reasons . . .

Thomas's understanding of habit gave the pastors theological language with which they could articulate the care of health as faithful rather than selfish and as a lifestyle that includes the whole person—mind, emotions, and body.

Pastors also resonated with Aquinas's understanding of the practice of health as having a mean between two extremes. The word "balance" came up repeatedly as pastors described both the clerical propensity toward self-denial, and the need to model effective self-care for parishioners. Aquinas's incorporation of Aristotelian thought of "mean" in health practices provided them with a way to conceive of a healthy balance in lives filled with extremes.

Lastly, clergy robustly endorsed Aquinas's teaching that habits of health orient to a larger *telos* of love of God and neighbor. Several interviewees affirmed that understanding health practices as directed toward flourishing would help "sell" clergy on the significance of care of their physical health; one pastor stated that if she understood getting on the treadmill as also being a spiritual discipline, it gives such a practice more weight. Another admitted that before CHI when he was overweight, he wasn't flourishing in ministry and had no fullness of God in life. When he started exercising and losing weight, he gained energy and zest for ministry again. Not only did he feel immensely better, but his relationships with parishioners and his ability to pastor improved—a living witness to the practice of habits of health as ultimately directed to greater service of God rather than self. In reflecting on Aquinas's understanding of habit as oriented to greater love, pastors said:

> I take Aquinas to mean that we aren't just pursuing goals . . . the mission is to know God and love others. One of our purposes is to care for the body—without which we can't love and know God and others as some disembodied mist. The goals of losing weight are not bad—but do they serve the purposes above them? To lose weight means you have greater energy during the day, your insulin sugar equation is better, you are more alert during the day. It makes a lot of sense—the idea of habit. To set a goal and be motivated by a higher purpose . . . Thomas' understanding of habit is very much on target based on what works for me and the stewardship of what we have been given. I have been given this body to use for God's glory and for the love of God and love of neighbor. If you only do it (habits of health) for a certain goal, like weight loss or heart rate, once you achieve it you won't keep it—unless you know it is to your benefit and everyone else's.

One interviewee, in reflecting on the practice of habits of health as ending in a greater love of God, neighbor, and self, remarked that Jesus's commandment to love oneself isn't "gushy" stuff, but that "love for self can be very pointed and hard." The difficulty for pastors in cultivating habits of health indicates how hard such practices are; Aquinas himself understands that the nurture of habits of virtue isn't for the fainthearted and requires all of ones' being. Yet, the true flourishing revealed upon the faithful practice of good habits makes such effort all worthwhile. Next, we'll examine the testimony of pastors as they reflect on how their new practices of health out of CHI changed their lives.

How We've Changed: Reflections on New Habits

New Practices Result in Greater Health

Out of their year long experience with CHI many of the interviewees now sustain healthier habits. More of the clergy have regular exercise habits and practice better nutrition with more fruits, vegetables, and home-cooked meals. Aside from the almost expected practices of better diet and exercise, clergypersons also described a regular practice of spiritual retreat, preparations for retirement, and counseling sessions. With all of

PART TWO—Habits of Health in Christian Community

their new habits, clergy felt healthier, happier, and that they were better pastors. One pastor's remarks indicate the link between greater physical health and a more balanced approach to her work:

> I learned in my meals not just to eat healthy but to make them smaller meals several times a day, rather than pigging out at night. I learned to sleep more and rest more. I take half days off now and I take a vacation every year . . . I thought I just had to keep on keeping on in ministry . . . I am not indispensible. With getting my weight off I am able to get out and do more. I am better able to handle people who are ill, sick, and grieving. I can be with them but not swallow up everything and take it with me emotionally . . .

Another pastor who was physically healthy focused his CHI resources upon cultivating greater emotional and spiritual health, and echoed the statements of other interviewees when he commented on his appreciation for CHI's broad latitude for the care of health. He stated:

> Extreme stress had become a way of life . . . In dealing with stress (with CHI) I uncovered issues about self-destruction in communicating and self-protective measures . . . Those are the things we worked on in CHI—on the emotional and spiritual side of things . . . I'm very grateful that the initiative allowed us the breadth to deal with that.

By practicing what Karl Barth called the Christian duty to live the healthiest life possible the clergy did indeed become more whole in body and in soul.[23] As the interviewees habituated their bodies with better nutrition and exercise, their souls became more conformed to God—just as Aquinas's anthropology indicates.

Greater Flourishing

Aside from growing habits of health clergy also mentioned more vitality within their lives. The habits provided an impetus for overall change; like Aquinas's theology teaches, these pastors embody the truth that quotidian habits transform us into more loving and gracious people. Several pastors testified to larger renovations in their lives due to better health practices:

---

23. Barth, *Doctrine of Creation*.

> I am engaged, not dismissive. I would be there and here and wouldn't listen before . . . I am more alive, more engaged, less fatigued, I'm sleeping more and better, I am more alert when I wake up . . . The office manager said "We like this Reverend better." I didn't realize I had alienated some people and maybe was vacant. I would sit a lot in the chair and wonder when I could go home and eat. Now I feel alive. Engaged is my word.
>
> I am a whole lot more patient and open and not so critical of myself. I have good boundaries because I realize that I have to take care of me; I can't take care of them if I don't care for me. The 95-year old (in my congregation) asks if I'm taking time off and taking care of myself—spending time with my husband . . . Boundaries are one of the best things I've learned from CHI . . .

In yet another confirmation of Aquinas's moral strategy, the pastors affirmed that positive changes in exercise/diet habits sculpted them into more lovely, more vibrant human beings who were better pastors for having taken time to work on themselves.

The Significance of "Accountability" Relationships

The interviewees made a striking number of references to learning through CHI of the imperative of having strong collegial relationships with other clergy. Though most knew before CHI of the importance of having good friendships, CHI helped this aspect of health to stand out in bold relief.

> I think CHI has forced me to recognize the lone ranger effect. I had heard about it before, but always thought "that's not me." Then to look and see that maybe I was trying to do everything myself instead of relying on others. The (CHI) coaching process helped me to open up to another clergy colleague about what is going on . . . I tend to not want another person to know about me because that person might become a DS (district superintendent). We have a fear mentality as clergy rather than trusting and helping one another . . . I didn't realize I was pursuing that path. (CHI) has allowed me to be more open with others. I need a support group that is outside of family that is going through similar experiences.
>
> My relationships with friends has become a lot more scary and vulnerable and real—That could have to do with trying to pray more. The Clergy Health Initiative coach helped me to key into my need to talk with people and be in contact with friends.

PART TWO—Habits of Health in Christian Community

> At first (in ministry) I isolated myself. The health coach helped me to identify community outside the congregation.

Not only did friendships with other clergy provide necessary emotional and spiritual support through the extraordinary challenges of ministry, but these relationships also offered accountability for health practices. The interviewees, who mentioned the word "accountability" repeatedly, felt that a strong communion of fellow clergy could hold them to their commitments to be faithful in care of their body, mind, and spirit. One clergyperson described her experience with her "accountability group":

> I would encourage anyone coming into the ministry to have an accountability partner—someone to ask "how is it with your soul?" I have three girlfriends in a covenant group and we meet once a month—and lots of it is accountability. If I tell them I'm struggling to be with my family, my husband, or shortchanging an area of life, they are going to ask me about it. We function better with accountability. I lost thirty pounds with Weight Watchers because I had accountability . . . The (accountability) person can't be the DS—it has to be fellow clergy—someone who will listen and say to you, "you need to reconsider and take vacation time."

For clergy, a communion of friends provides vital support in the sustenance of habits of health. Due to being the leader of the congregation, their accountability for their practices generally cannot come from their church community, but rather from a circle of fellow pastors. As one clergyperson put it, "by reaching out to others I come to know how I can be myself." Such sentiments affirm what Aquinas wrote about friendship in the *Summa*, namely that we practice morality in community and these relationships form us and sustain us in the ongoing work of cultivating health.

An Ongoing Journey

With honesty and vulnerability the clergy admitted that they hadn't arrived yet at optimal health practices after a year in the pilot program. They described their habits of health as a journey of sanctification in which they would always have ongoing work. One pastor stated that the CHI program "caused me to think again or more about how maintaining my body is a part of sanctification." Though CHI certainly made a difference in the lives of all of the interviewees, some had life transformation while others felt it had just given them new insight or information—and others admitted to ongoing struggles to overcome health issues.

> I know that my weight can be better . . . I want to be a disciplined person yet it is the hardest thing in the world. Someone is dying and in the hospital—how do I make more time? I don't know if I can do anything more efficiently. Something's gotta give. I can't figure it out yet. I don't know how to make more time . . .

Another clergyperson admitted in the interview question about what changes he had made in his health since CHI:

> Not many, unfortunately. I know I shouldn't should on myself. (CHI) had the potential to be life-changing. Other things I've been dealing with have proved more distracting. The major change is that the family does more biking together. I would still like to get back into an exercise routine. I have struggled with cigarette smoking and other addictive habits that in stressful times I return to . . . it was a great program but it didn't have any life-long changing effect.

These clergy's truthful admittances of the ongoing struggle of maintaining healthy habits, even after the incredible support and resources of the Clergy Health Initiative, indicates what a great challenge real change in health habits remains for people. In his discussions on the will, reason, and habit, Aquinas also affirms that permanent change remains extraordinarily difficult for human beings. Healthcare remains a lifelong journey, and some of the clergy were in a better place to make changes in their lives when they began the pilot program than others. Those not ready to make drastic changes would have been in the precontemplation stage before the program began, while those who did undertake new habits would have been in the contemplation stage. Thomas's theology of the multilayered action of the will offers further support for clergy who are not sufficiently habituated into lives of health.

A Healthier Church

Even with all of the hindrances to health for clergy from their local church and from the larger United Methodist System, several mentioned how their local church supported them through the pilot program. In one church a Boy Scout transformed a dank, unused room into a fitness

PART TWO—Habits of Health in Christian Community

center for his Eagle Scout project. One of the pastors of that church—a church that had lost previous pastors due to heart attacks—stated that

> The congregation is proud that I am taking time for self-care ... The SPRC (staff-parish relations committee) said to me "you take care of you (name omitted) and your health. You cannot be present with us if you are unhealthy."

Another pastor said that her church was proud of her when she did take time to work out and that they had done a study on the book by Stephanie Paulsell called *Honoring the Body*.

Beyond their local church, pastors envisioned change on a broader scope within the United Methodist Church. Out of their experience with CHI, pastors felt convicted that the entire church needed to become a system in which health is supported and part of the fabric of the Methodist culture.

> I have colleague who is afraid of working out (for fear of what his congregation would think/do). The man captures what we need to do as a denomination. We need to move the (health) issue from an aside to an integral aspect of how we do our denomination. We need to make it an expectation to take care of ourself—as part of how we "do business." Until it becomes integrated into denominational structures and the *Discipline* ... we will have to have extra courage to press ahead with things like this.
>
> Health needs to become part of the fabric of the denomination, part of going through seminary and the denomination so that this (health) is part of who you are as a pastor—where this (health) becomes the norm in churches and PPSRCs. (so that chuches say) "Yes, our pastor works out. We are Methodists. This is what we do." I remember when I used to work for the police department and the police officers were donut eaters. The younger generation came in with police officers who worked out as part of their job. The department built a work-out area and gym. It (exercising) became a part of what you did, and as you did this you became a better police officer. There should be incentives for pastors to join the Y in districts instead of just eating together all the time. The PPSRC should be like "yes, you are doing this! (exercising). (Exercise) should be something you feel shameful about, but rather realize that you are a better pastor because you do this.

The clergy longed for a church culture in which it is expected that they take care of their health, instead of one in which workaholism is often affirmed and encouraged in order to climb higher on the appointment ladder. They articulated a desire to call the United Methodist Church into greater faithfulness in regards to the care of health and wellbeing—yet they also felt disempowered to be able to enact any cultural change themselves. They hoped that CHI, and other programs like it, might help a largely dysfunctional church when it comes to health matters learn to become a system that nurtures the wellbeing of its leaders, rather than eroding it. The clergy cast a vision for a church that would truly embody its theology, and support healthy habits as integral to Christian life and witness. Such a vision could be sustained and supported by the thought of Aquinas, whose theology of habit reminds the church to be incarnational and provides a pathway to do so. Aquinas's thought affirms the pastors' admonition that "health needs to become part of who we are as a church;" Thomistic habit explicitly offers that we are what we do. For the clerical interviewees, the United Methodist Church needs to dramatically shift to doing more health practices if it is to ever transform into a healthier denomination.

Discussion of the Results

Good Theology of the Body Doesn't Necessarily Lead to Health

All of the interviewees articulated a theology in which the body is worthy of care and scripture affirms the body as good and holy. Yet even with a clear understanding of the body as gift and of the call to tend to the "temple of the Holy Spirit" many of the pastors were doing poor work of caring for their bodies before the CHI pilot program. Of course, in their defense one could point to all of the hindrances described above that inhibit pastors' ability to care for their health. However, through the intervention of CHI all of the clergy made changes in their health practices—some quite dramatic and transformational. Even those who didn't have a life-changing experience with CHI had made at least small, positive changes in their practices. Why did these clergy, with thoughtful theologies of body, not practice good healthcare before CHI, and why was CHI so successful in prompting change in habits that theology alone couldn't do?

To begin with, theology divorced from action perhaps isn't true belief. Such a dichotomy represents a core of Martin Luther's argument that faith must not be separated from works.[24] To divide theology from ethics denotes a fallacy perpetuated from the Enlightenment. CHI, though perhaps not intentionally in the pilot program, brought together these pastors' embedded theologies of the body with a whole set of practices, including regular physician visits, covenant groups, and health coaching. CHI nudged what the pastors thought about health into actual practice. CHI served as a catalyst to move participants from a stage of contemplation into preparation and action. As one pastor stated, "You have to put ethics with health—it's basically the same thing." CHI helped these interviewees to do just that.

Secondly, the pastors' theology of the body, even with its goodness, wasn't that well-developed. None of the interviewees grew up in churches in which the Christian responsibility to care for health was taught. Each entered into seminary with this catechetical weakness, and the seminary where most of them went didn't strengthen them in practices of health.[25] Most of them didn't receive teaching that the care of their bodies/health was worth whatever sacrifice of work/productivity it required. Within the demanding rigor of their theological education they weren't taught of the Wesleyan emphasis on holistic health, nor that service to the church didn't demand the sacrifice of their health. Without a rich theology and a seminary education that affirmed the care of their well-being, the pastors were ill-equipped to handle the rigors of ministry and thus many quickly offered up any care of themselves in the swamping needs of their congregations.

The Theology of Aquinas and Wesley Is Vital

Wesley's holistic understanding of salvation and Aquinas's theology of habit offer essential development to the clergy's existing understanding of the good of the body. First, John Wesley's theology and practice of

---

24. For a fuller description of Luther's argument on this point. See Luther, *Freedom of a Christian*.

25. Several of the clergy articulated that health wasn't taught in seminary. After nine years at this same institution as a Master of Divinity and then doctoral student I would corroborate that the seminary pays an inordinate amount of attention to intellectual formation, then some to spiritual formation, and little to no attention to students' physical/mental/emotional formation for life in ministry.

healthcare provides an affirming heritage for these United Methodist clergy. From the founder of the "people called Methodists" the pastors can derive rich teaching on the significance of personal and communal health for their congregrations—and for themselves.

Secondly, Aquinas provides life-giving insights for health—namely that the practice of habits of health leads to greater flourishing for the pastors and their congregations. By caring from themselves, the pastors can then better love God and those whom they serve. The vibrant demeanor of clergy who had lost weight/practiced exercise/nurtured new habits testifies to the truth of Aquinas's thought. Aquinas's understanding of habits as directing people to a life of greater virtue and love provides the invaluable insight for clergy that the care of oneself is "worth it." The interviewees resonated strongly with healthcare being motivated by a higher purpose/*telos* and overwhelming appreciated a theology that can sustain them in their hard-won disciplines of health. A Thomist hermeneutic of healthcare supports the practice of good habits, while at the same time describing the beautiful transformations that come out of such practice.

Virtue

Many of the interviewees articulated that they were changed persons because of CHI; they are now more patient, kind, engaged, and alive to their congregations. Without using the language of the cardinal virtues they nonetheless demonstrated that they had become more virtuous people. Out of any virtue, it seems that the interviewees learned temperance. Whereas before CHI they ate too much or exercised too little, after CHI they learned to eat and exercise in the mean. For others, they learned to not have excess stress or to work in the extreme. Person after person described a life in which temperance governed their relationships to their bodies and health.

Of course, where temperance exists there must also be prudence. Through participation in CHI the pastors learned to train their reason rightly. They learned better discernment about their health and came to "see" rightly how important their wellbeing is for their life and ministry. The clergy now practice better judgment about their health, which results in happier, more fulfilled lives and ministry.

The interviewees also practiced the virtue of courage. Some of them had to go against their parish's culture to take time to exercise, and had

PART TWO—Habits of Health in Christian Community

to delicately refuse unhealthy food offered to them at church gatherings and potlucks. In pursuing a new habit, each pastor had to be steadfast in the midst of enormous barriers and hindrances to health. In a vocation replete with constant interruptions they had to stand their ground and persevere in practices of health. The clergy had to be brave in order to be healthy.

None of the clergy made connections of their practices of health to larger issues of injustice in regards to health in their communities. Yet, the persecution that some clergy endure from their congregations means that they themselves are often victims of injustice. In taking a stand for themselves and practicing the care of their health the clergy are making a stand for justice. Hopefully out of their CHI experience clergy will become more attentive to issues of injustice that perpetuate disease within their communities.

United Methodist Church Needs to Address Health

The honest complaints of these pastors about their church's harm to their health needs to be taken seriously by bishops and district superintendents. Of course one motivating factor, mentioned by a couple of clergy, is the skyrocketing cost of health insurance for clergy. Yet, rather than admonishing the clergy to "practice better self-care," conferences, including General Conference, must do the difficult and courageous work of changing dysfunctional aspects of the Methodist system which contribute to poor clergy health—not only because of the "bottom line" in regards to health insurance, but also because good health is faithful and enables pastors to be more effective.

One of those problematic aspects remains the appointment system—a system that has become burdened by its promise of guarantee, interchurch politics, and linkage to compensation packages. All of these factors lead to young or inexperienced pastors being placed in difficult, often dysfunctional churches with low pay. Older pastors with greater longevity receive urban/suburban appointments with greater salaries—even if they are incompetent. As Bishop Peter Storey of South Africa (where compensation is not tied to appointment and all pastors are paid equitable amounts) says, the American church must disconnect salary and church size in order to be faithful. One could say that the church needs to do this also in order for clergy to be healthy.

Another aspect, even harder to change than the appointment system, is a church culture than condones workaholism and doesn't affirm the practice of diet and exercise as important—and where unhealthy food tends to be ubiquitously present. Such a cultural change requires courageous teaching from the episcopacy and churches open to new ways of being. When the church displays insufficient habituation in the virtuous life, Thomas's teaching on habit reminds the church to orient to a *telos* of God and lives of flourishing.

Conclusion

The experience of the clergy in CHI proves that Aquinas's theology of habit does have real traction in the lives of Christians. The Thomist account of health as moral action describes how the clergy were able to become more wholesome people. The pastors' adoption of new practices of health changed their lives; for those who were dedicated, these changes led to transformation. Not only were weight lost and blood pressures lowered, but people became more loving to their parishoners and more present to their families and themselves. They lived into new vitality—and their relationships with God and others improved because of it. In effect, these CHI participants lived into *eudaimonia*. From new habits of health they entered into true flourishing—just as Thomas teaches.

10

Word Made Flesh

Introduction to Word Made Flesh and Community Care

IN ADDITION TO THE STRESS, POOR HEALTH, AND HIGH DEMANDS WITH which American clergy wrestle, missionaries must also struggle with a wide array of tropical diseases (such as malaria), unsafe water, contaminated or scarce food, lack of access to physical exercise, and volatile governments.[1] American missionaries in other lands often lack access to basic healthcare services, work in languages other than their mother tongue of English (inherently stressful and exhausting), and raise their own children in daunting circumstances.[2] Missionaries' face even more barriers than clergy in any attempt to cultivate practices of health. I wanted to explore one missionary organization, and their efforts to overcome multiple barriers in order to nurture their members to flourishing; I settled upon Word Made Flesh.

Founded in 1991 as a non-profit organization, Word Made Flesh (WMF) is an evangelical Christian ministry that serves the most vulnerable of the world's population, including destitute children and women forced to be commercial sex slaves. The first missionary went to Chennai, India in 1994 where WMF opened a children's home devoted to pediatric

---

1. Lange et al., "Missionary Health," 332–38. This article indicates the high levels of malaria and hepatitis B among sub-Saharan missionaries and notes the need for attention to mental health and comprehensive health services for missionaries working in destitute, disease-ridden areas.

2. Dwelle, "Inadequate Basic Preventative Health Measures," 733–37. This article discussed the inadequate health services for missionary children, their low rates of immunizations, and their exposure to untreated water and produce.

AIDS care.³ Since then WMF has established communities of service in ten countries in Asia, Latin America, Europe, and Africa. WMF's vision is to "serve Jesus among the most vulnerable of the world's poor. This calling is realized as a prophetic ministry for, and an incarnational, holistic mission among the poor" in urban settings.⁴ In their work and service with women and children WMF upholds nine core values: intimacy, obedience, humility, community, service, simplicity, submission, brokenness, and suffering. With 60 U.S. based staff (in Omaha, NE) and over 200 employees worldwide WMF is now in its twentieth year of missional, communal service with the poor.

In 2004, after years of seeing staff burning out, getting sick, and neglecting personal health, the administration of WMF created the Community Care center to respond to the mental, physical, and spiritual health of its people and to contradict damaging dualisms found within evangelicalism.⁵ The Community Care Center, now staffed by two people based in Omaha, offers support and resources to tend to the health of missionaries on the field and U.S. based staff. The center offers orientation and pre-mission fieldwork training and provides a formation program for the first three years of a missionary's service.⁶ Community Care also provides connections to spiritual directors and mental health counselors, directs staff to medical care they can access in their area, offers support for vocational discernment, provides resources for staff entering into their sabbaticals after seven years of service and offers leaves of absence for staff.⁷ In instances of tragedy or significant staff transitions/

---

3. Word Made Flesh, "About WMF."

4. Word Made Flesh, "About WMF," see "Vision Statement."

5. Phileena Heurtz, co-director of Word Made Flesh. Interview, Feb. 15, 2010.

6. Silas West, director of Community Care for Word Made Flesh. Interview, July 18, 2010. The formation program was just being finalized and launched during the Staff Gathering in the summer of 2010. It consists of readings/books/articles required for the missionaries in orientation, pre-departure, and the first three years of service. The intent of the formation materials are to provide: "1. Personal growth and spiritual formation 2. A sense of uniform continuity and understanding of issues involved in ministry among the poor within the WMF community 3. Suggestions and insight to aid in applied ministry principles and concepts 4. Materials and ideas for discipleship, teaching, preaching, and other similar settings." Word Made Flesh, "Formation Materials," 3. In effect, the formation program serves as a "mini-seminary," training people from a wide variety of backgrounds in theology, missiology, spirituality, and personal care.

7. Ibid. WMF has published a sabbatical guide, which offers a description of sabbatical, the purpose of it, seven phases of it for WMF staffers, and reflections from the

PART TWO—Habits of Health in Christian Community

issues on the field, community care offers "critical incident debriefing" to support members through difficult changes. The Community Care Center affirms WMF's commitment to the whole person through vocational development, retreats, and contemplative prayer practices among its staff. In addition, each community in the mission setting has a person responsible for community care; he or she monitors and supports the health of individuals within that field.[8] After Community Care's six years in existence, leaders within WMF have noticed healthier function within the organization and positive growth among staff members.

Methodology

I collected data through personal interviews with American staff of Word Made Flesh while they were attending their triennial Gathering at the Lied Lodge in Nebraska in August 2010.[9] I conducted eighteen individual interviews; the gender distribution was six males and twelve females, which rather fairly reflects the gender make-up of WMF employees.[10] The interview questions consisted of ten structured questions; the questions asked about the person's history and work with WMF, participation in community care or wellness programs of WMF, and reflections upon

---

community on experiences of sabbatical. Phileena Heuertz, "Sabbatical Guide." Leaves of absence have been offered to staff for the death of a significant family member, for the birth/adoption of a child, for miscarriage, and for health reasons.

8. WMF has published a health guide for its missionaries that affirms WMF's commitment to good health and holism for staff who serve in countries with prevalent disease and poverty. It describes requirements for staff to receive vaccinations/malaria prophylaxis, physician health check-ups, and travel/health insurance as well as recommendations for nurturing physical, emotional, and mental health. It is required reading in the formation program. Curless, Haley, and Heuertz, "Health Guide."

9. After initially planning on recruiting participants before the Gathering by email, the co-director of WMF, a staff liason, and I decided to recruit by a sign-up form and an announcement at the beginning of the Gathering, when everyone was assembled and had a better sense of what times they might have free for an interview. On the first evening of the gathering and at subsequent corporate times I passed around a sign-up sheet and eventually received eighteen responses; the director and co-director also informally encouraged people to sign up for the interviews.

10. Four of the interviewees, including the director and co-director and the director of Community Care, are based in the US; fourteen of the staffers are based internationally, representing communities in Sierra Leone, Romania, Argentina, Peru, Romania, India, Moldova, and Brazil. Seven of the international missionaries interviewed serve as directors of Community Care within their field. One of the interviewees is Romanian, and married to an American Romanian-based missionary.

any changes in their life and health as a result of said participation.[11] Out of this field research key domains emerged on barriers to health for missionaries, a practical theology of health, and new habits missionaries and WMF developed out of Community Care—all of which will be explored below. I'll conclude with some comparisons of WMF and the Clergy Health Initiative discussed earlier and how both of these institutions ended with greater flourishing.

Hindrances to Healthcare for Staff

Many of the barriers faced by the missionaries correlated with the United Methodist clergy; both populations work in demanding service contexts. However the degree of hindrances to health for the missionaries appeared even more intense than for the clergy; the staff of WMF had more to overcome in order to nurture transformative habits. I'll now describe those obstructions to good health, describing first personal and then institutional obstacles.

Negative or Absent Formation in Health from Churches of Childhood

Many of the missionaries, unlike the clergy, had explicitly negative teachings about the body in their churches of childhood. Several used the term "repressive" to describe their church's catechesis on embodiment. One staffer said that in his Church of Christ congregation the body was seen

---

11. A couple of questions were altered during the course of the interviews and one was deleted. If I could do the interviews again, I would add the theological and Aquinas questions from my interviews with the clergy. The interviews reached the point of redundancy before all eighteen were completed, but out of gratitude for their graciousness in volunteering time and because of the different contexts in which people served I continued through all the sign-ups. The interviews lasted 30-45 minutes and the Duke University Institutional Review Board approved the study. The interviews were recorded and verbatim notes were taken during the interviews. I did experience technological issues with my recording device during the interviews, resulting in a loss of some material. In addition to conducting interviews, I also taught the WMF employees yoga twice a day, ate meals with them, and participated in worship and other programs. Therefore the interviewees viewed me as someone committed to health through yoga, and we developed relationships during the course of the ten days I was there. My participation in the community's life during the Gathering could influence the data analysis.

as guilty and any teaching on the body would have been against the body. Females within the WMF population definitely had damaging influences:

> I was repressed growing up in regards to bodily expression. I grew up in a conservative church where dancing wasn't allowed. The body was always referred to in regards to sexual sin. Outward appearance was still valued; (for females) there were no pants and I wasn't allowed to wear makeup or earrings. How I perceived the body was repressive . . .

> I grew up in a Bible-believing, fundamental/evangelical tradition. People were uncomfortable with movement. There was no holding of hands and no clapping. I remember having to wear nylons as a kid; all girls had to wear skirts and nylons. There was general discomfort with women's bodies. *True Love Waits* was really big . . . there was to be no kissing and virginity was huge. It was considered a badge of honor not to kiss anyone; you were to have no sexual needs or desires . . .

A few WMF staffers mentioned dualisms about the body/spirit that they imbibed from their church of origin. In a conservative, small church of Wesleyan Armenian tradition one interviewee experienced a "real separation of what is spiritual and what isn't" . . . there was a real categorization and split. You couldn't be a whole person." Another said that in her congregational church there was a real dichotomy between body and soul: "you learned of the health of the soul but there was no focus on the body. The health of the body is what you went to the doctor for." Through such dualistic teachings WMF staffers learned that care of the spirit was more important and valuable that care of the body.

A high number of WMF employees grew up as "preacher's kids" in which their father (always the father) pastored the church. Some described a pressure to be "perfect" in behavior and appearance and the toll that took on them emotionally and physically.

> In my adolescence I was in a missionary church; my dad was the pastor. I had intense pressure to be perfect and that related to my body. Yet all church gatherings revolved around food—and there was nothing healthy there. They had lots of pig roasts. I came out thinking that I needed to be perfect . . . so I started in 7th and 8th grade to experiment with not eating . . .

Another "preacher's kid" mentioned seeing how her mother's mental and emotional health was neglected and the church provided no support for healthcare (physical or emotional) for the pastor's family. A pastor's son echoed such sentiments; his church of origin felt that wellness was a luxury and austerity should reign. Following the rules of the church meant denying any care of oneself and minimalizing emotional needs.

Other interviewees mentioned the complete absence of any discussion of or teaching upon physical wellness or the body. The one staffer raised in the United Methodist Church echoed the experiences of the clergy I interviewed when she said, "The body wasn't addressed in our church. It wasn't talked about. It wasn't a priority." Another person, who said she was raised in a very conservative church, commented that:

> We did devotionals, read the bible, and prayed. I don't remember any talk about physical wellness or a connection between that and spiritual wellness. Health in its fullness was not emphasized growing up.

A staffer who grew up in a California town on the coast remarked that the absence of any teaching on health in his church was remarkable, given that they lived in a beach community with a large surfing subculture in which health was a priority for many people. Yet another staff person said about wellness and the body in the church, "It was not a topic; it wasn't discussed. Mainstream adolescent messages from high school had more of an impact." Thus, by lack of any catechesis or teaching on the body in Christian lives, the missionaries learned that the body wasn't as significant or as important as their soul. With so many staffers with either a negative or absent formation on the body immersed in incredibly difficult work, the next barrier to good health comes as no surprise—the willingness to sacrifice your body for the sake of service to others.

Sacrifice Is What Is Required of You

Several of the senior missionary staff felt that they needed to live a life of sacrifice when they first arrived on the field. They experienced an internal pressure to live as the people around them did—trying to emulate the children/youth of their setting who were trying to survive on the streets. One person said, "when I first came (to the mission field) I didn't take care of myself in identification with the people. I thought that self-martyrdom was good." Others described their initial time of service this way:

> Looking back on my first days in WMF I think of how I wanted to have God's heart for service . . . and there was some

> immaturity there. I found worth in what I did, and going to all lengths meant damaging my own personal body.
>
> When we first moved to Peru I lost weight... I felt that I needed to sacrifice. I thought that in caring for others I was not to care for myself. It was my own perception of who I thought I should be...

The desire of WMF staff to lead what they thought was a faithful, sacrificial life led to some devastating health consequences for a couple of missionaries, to burn-out and departure from the mission field for others, and to a complete lack of flourishing for all who practiced such ascetic self-denial.

Health Challenges in Field Settings

Missionaries mentioned a litany of diseases they had suffered in their countries of service, from sinus infections to gastrointestinal issues to emotional exhaustion. Due to the nature of their work in developing countries, many of which lack adequate sanitation and are rife with disease from malaria to stomach bugs, WMF staff experience copious levels of sickness and disease. In addition, "WMF staff serve among people who, due to poverty, suffer from a high burden of disease even compared to the majority of the population in that country."[12] An interviewee who lives at 13,800 feet in Bolivia mentioned how tiring work is at such altitude and how the altitude wears on your body. A missionary in Brazil noted how difficult it was at first to find ingredients for cooking healthy meals. Another mentioned that in his setting no gym facilities existed—or even safe places to go for a jog. A missionary in Peru noted that even discussions of stress and trauma feel like a luxury in a place in which people operate in complete survival mode and don't have opportunities to rest and process their lives. This whole bricolage of descriptions of challenging life/work settings depicts why sickness easily enters into the lives of WMF staffers.

The Nature of the Work

Interviewees described their work as making relationships with the most vulnerable populations in the world. Many WMFers work with street

---

12. Curless, Haley, and Heuertz, "Health Guide," 7.

Word Made Flesh

children in the slums of large cities or support women as they leave enslavement in the sex trade. They run discipleship programs, community centers, and handicraft businesses. Such work taxes people emotionally and physically. Missionaries who work with children in Romania said:

> The nature of the work has taken a toll . . . coming into close contact with deep suffering in the lives of children is like a secondary trauma. It's very difficult emotionally . . .

> It is overwhelming many times. I see many problems as I offer therapy. I absorb people's energy—I really sense their energy and take it in. If I'm tired I can't control as well how much I absorb. I carry the burdens of people . . . I have had to learn to give things to the Lord—If I neglect that it's not good for me.

In addition, not only do individual missionaries get weary from the work, but an entire WMF community can become fatigued from the suffering and struggle around them. A staffer in Peru described how the WMF native Peruvian staff needed lots of support and help as they worked with their own people, but noted that such work is "hard in places where the church is thin with energy because of constant helping." When a whole community becomes too "thin" from constant service, health problems are sure to follow.

Work without Rhythm

Lastly, missionaries noted their own internal drives toward workaholism without any kind of holy rhythm. In their positions of service and in the face of overwhelming need they felt they must constantly work—especially if they were starting a new field (i.e. setting up a new place in the world for WMF to create community and serve) or beginning their first term of service for WMF. A missionary in Romania admitted that "I don't feel like I have the right balance . . . some of us are workaholics and I always feel like I'm not working hard enough." Another confessed that when she first arrived on the field she "ran herself ragged" and worked all of the time, finding it very difficult to set healthy rhythms. The struggle to find a healing and wholesome rhythm of life arose in many of the missionaries' interviews as they described lives of everpresent work and need.

PART TWO—Habits of Health in Christian Community

Institutional Barrier: Culture of "Sink or Swim"

The WMF staff was candid and honest in describing challenges to health due to their own organization's systems and way of being. Prior to the creation of Community Care in 2004 the staff described a culture in which people weren't taking care of themselves and were wearing themselves out. A staffer described the culture this way: "people were camping all the time. No one could pursue their own interests or even join a gym." A missionary who started in 2002 said WMF was "a culture of sink or swim, you either make it or you don't."

To WMF's credit, all of the interviewees with longevity in the organization noted what a drastic transformation has occurred in the organization since the inception of Community Care in 2004. This cultural change will be described in more detail in the section below on "new habits." However, the point to make here is that for many years WMF had a culture in which staffers felt wellbeing wasn't central and physical/emotional/mental health was largely ignored.

Institutional Barrier: Conflict Management

Administrative staff (based in Omaha) were quite honest and open in admitting that their organization struggled with conflict, especially in the area of "saying goodbye." The director of WMF confessed that WMF doesn't let go of people well, often blames them when they leave, and creates more grief. Another Omaha-based staffer spoke about the transient nature of the community and the struggle WMF has with allowing people to move out of the organization.

> We are not good at letting people leave. Close friends in WMF have left and they didn't feel supported. If the vocation is outside of the organization we are not good at validating. If they discover something we didn't want then we say how dare you. We have a high attrition rate because we take everything hard and put it together. We have to raise our own support, live in community, and partner with the people of the culture. We draw people with intense personalities and have lots of overachievers without any infrastructure to sustain people before Community Care.

The director of Community Care acknowledged that WMF needs to work on communication skills, particularly when divisions exist among staff. He described the enormous amount of loss the community

Word Made Flesh

endures—from the abuse of women to the murder of children—and the need to process and communicate well about those griefs. He stated:

> The (WMF) culture doesn't give the permission to grieve well, which then festers in insidious ways in the (WMF) culture. We have lots of losses and we bring our own losses into the mix. Being stuck in lots of loss and grief leads to tensions and unresolved issues. We need to be able to communicate well through that. We need to create more stable communities even as people come and go.

Institutional Barrier: Administrative Burden

Missionaries on the field, particularly senior staff, described their responsibilities as encompassing a profuse amount of administration. Some spoke of desk work, which kept them from actually being with the children/youth/women they were there to serve. Staff from different fields commented:

> I came on the field idealistic and starry-eyed. I didn't think I would have to jump through legal hopes and form a board. Sometimes the work is not about being with the people we are serving...

> WMF has a top-down leadership that requires rather than (nurtures) self-initative. It's a hard line to walk... WMF is being authoritative so that people don't fail. There may be some passive aggressiveness and fear of being too authoritative because of the culture of the organization...

One senior staffer mentioned that WMF had gaps in support to senior staff on the field—while at the same time requiring a great deal from them. WMF's administrative burden appeared to add more stress and less job satisfaction to the interviewees, which in turn negatively impacts staffers' health.

The Manna Question—What Is It?

In conducting eighteen interviews I received an enormous variety of responses for the question asking for a description of and experiences of Community Care. A few talked exclusively of sabbaticals, while several mentioned prayer practices and others noted personal retreats. Such a

PART TWO—Habits of Health in Christian Community

cornucopia of replies could indicate the depth and breadth of Community Care's services in WMF—and to an extent that is true. However, even after doing eighteen interviewees I struggled to put together a clear picture of Community Care. Several of the missionaries, particularly those serving as community care liasons in their field, mentioned that Community Care is constantly growing and expanding, and they are eager to learn what it offers. Everyone seemed very excited and grateful that it existed, but wasn't exactly sure what "it" was. Below are some statements from missionaries in the field who serve as Community Care liasons.

> I'm becoming passionate about Community Care and trying to learn what is being offered to us. There is a biannual health check by a doctor, formation practices, spiritual retreats, staff retreats, materials about contemplative prayer practices, strength tests, spiritual disciplines, personality tests . . .

> Community Care is growing all the time. There are lots of debriefing resources, support for counselors/spiritual directors, resources for prayer practices, different retreat centers to go to, policies for sabbaticals, leave of absences, personal retreats, maternity leaves, critical incident debriefing . . . It would be great if Community Care could help us develop resources in our country of service and compile them so that we can easily access them—even a list of books like Michael Pollan's *In Defense of Food*.

> Community Care offers wellness programs. It focuses on the spiritual, emotional, and physical. We have to file board reports on how we are doing. It helps to create healthy rhythms, communally and individually.

Certainly these staffers don't contradict each other and several mentioned similar things. Yet a coherent vision and understanding of the scope of Community Care seemed to be lacking. Given the relatively nascent nature of the organization (Community Care was launched in 2004) and its ongoing expansion of services, some variation in understanding of its role isn't surprising. Some WMF staffers may not be participating in and receiving the benefits of Community Care because they don't know what is available to them. Greater awareness of its offerings among staff and a clear, consistent message of Community Care's purpose would ensure greater access to its services among staff, and would strengthen an institutional culture in which people commonly care for their health.

Lack of Pastoral Leadership

Several of the missionaries yearned for more pastoral care within WMF. Many mentioned how they had felt cared for by Phileena Heuertz, the co-director of WMF, during times of crisis or tragedy in their lives. However, staffers also felt that a person (s) trained in pastoral care could be of great service to their communities in their fields of service.

> Something really missing among us is pastoring. Our leaders aren't trained as pastors and aren't exactly pastoral . . . It (not having pastors) has been something really challenging—(pastoring) is something that could be utilized more. Phileeena has a pastoral heart but she can't be in all places at all times . . . we need people to guide us through scriptural truths, but we don't always have those people in place.

Another staffer admitted that pastoral leadership within the framework of Community Care is missing within WMF.

> The framework is there, but there is a lack of staff to support the framework and commitments to the community. (This gap) goes across the board in all communities. There are just not people there who have the time to do it (offer pastoral care) . . .

Without pastoral leadership and care within WMF's field communities staffers feel like they experience a gap in their spiritual life and growth.

Summary of Hindrances to Health

With heavy administrative burdens, poor conflict management, ambiguity about what Community Care is, and a workaholic culture WMF missionaries constantly endure compromises to their wellbeing. When all these institutional burdens combine with personal obstacles (negative catechesis on the body, sacrificial orientations, disease prevalence, and extraordinarily challenging work) it's no wonder that the WMF staff struggled with poor health in multiple dimensions of their lives. Like for the clergy, Aquinas's theology of habit acknowledges the difficult burdens the missionaries face, while at the same time offering a pathway into a better life. Thomas's offering of health as a virtuous practice encourages these missionaries to have faith that all challenges can be overcome in order to grow into closer life with God.

PART TWO—Habits of Health in Christian Community

Theology of Wellbeing

Just like the clergy, the missionaries forged a surprisingly robust and healthy theology—even as they lived with ailing health. Through personal and WMF-recommended reading as well as life in the crucible of ministry with the vulnerable, WMF staffers developed a practical theology—without any formal seminary training.

Unlike the interviews with the United Methodist clergy, I didn't ask the missionaries explicitly about their understanding of a theology of the body.[13] However, out of questions on their relationship with God in connection to practices of wellness I was able to cull a few theological themes within WMF. All of the staffers seemed well acquainted with the lifestyle celebrations (intimacy, obedience, humility, community, service, simplicity, submission, brokenness, and suffering), which serve as theological touchstones for the community. The themes delineated below affirm the theological commitments of the organization while at the same time reflecting a true practical theology from those immersed in the arduous work of loving Jesus's most vulnerable children.

Learning the True Self

WMF places an emphasis on active contemplation, in which spiritual practices merge with concrete service to those in need. Spiritual care comprises a major component of Community Care's responsibilities. One of the practices taught within WMF is centering prayer, in which a person sits in receptive silence for at least twenty minutes twice a day. Promulgated and taught by Father Thomas Keating, a Cistercian monk who resides at St. Benedict's Monastery in Snowmass, CO, centering prayer recovers a contemplative tradition in Christianity. Through faithful practice a person begins to shed "false" selves as he/she grows closer to God and becomes more the true person God created him/her to be.[14] The co-director, Phileena Heurtz, has deeply steeped herself in this practice, and imparts it to her WMF community

Among WMF staffers, those who described a prayer practice within their own daily rhythm also articulated that since their time in WMF

---

13. In retrospect I wish that I had! The WMF interviews came six months before the UM clergy interviews and before I had written on Aquinas's theology for the dissertation.

14. Keating, *Intimacy with God*.

they've discovered their true selves—language which comes out of Thomas Keating's work. Missionaries stated:

> As we are encouraged to know ourselves more, our interactions with others become more honest and vulnerable. As God heals the layers that healing translates into relationship with Him. We are known with all the messiness that we are. To feel okay being that person with other people is healing. We can be our true selves in front of God and everyone else.
>
> I value myself more now (after years of service with WMF). I understand that I am made in the image of God. This is a much healthier place to minister from. I'm more whole. Recognizing that I am made in the image of God is something beautiful. Now I am able to believe it and live it.

Out of their experiences with WMF and its emphasis on contemplation in the midst of an active life, these interviewees felt they had grown into more of their authentic selves—and in so doing grew closer to God and to others. Without being told of Aquinas's theology of habit, the WMF staff nonetheless affirmed Aquinas's insight that good habits (here habits of prayer) come to make us more fully who we are as individuals and draw us closer to God.[15]

God in the Suffering

WMF missionaries, who spend their lives working amid people enduring through extreme poverty, witness suffering daily. Rather than engaging in theodicy, however, the long-term missionaries testified to broadened understandings of God and God's presence with those who struggle for daily bread.

> My understanding of God has broadened in a good way (since working with WMF). It's more than what most Christians learn. I have a deeper recognition of faith. I used to wonder (when I first came on the field) "why doesn't God stop horrible things?" Now I see God is really present more than I see horrible things . . .
>
> (Service in WMF) has had a profound and intense effect. I've seen God through the stuff that is the most broken and painful. God is gracious and wants reconciliation. He is forgiving

---

15. Aquinas, *ST* I-II 49.2.

> through all the crap. I'm learning the immensity of God's love and grace . . . I'm learning to pray for the enemy (the perpetrators of abuse). It (service in WMF) has exploded my idea of who God is and what God wants. I've had times of exploded understanding of God's intention for the world.
>
> In two and a half years of employment with WMF, which is a prophetic community, I have a fuller understanding of who God is. I realize that Christianity is relationship with the poor . . . I'm becoming a broader thinking Christian. I think about how God relates to the rest of the world and not just my little world. I wrestle with suffering and abundance and where God is in all of this . . . I see God's desire to make all things new. I see the redemptive plan of the Bible. I see that (suffering) is not the end of the story. God is working a redemptive plan in the whole world . . . though at times it may be hard to see.
>
> I am learning how to lament, how to talk to God through the pain. I've realized that in the Garden of Eden there was joy, and pain entered with sin and anger. I know that our emotions are given by God to help us cope with the fallenness of the world. There will be times of grief, sadness, and pain . . . but learning about lamenting has been instrumental in me being able to continue on the field. It comes back to healing . . . now I am able to talk to God about pain . . .

Through their immersion in the grit of destitute poverty while at the same time practicing love and compassion, the staff of WMF developed a practical theology of suffering. In this theology, spun out of the crucible of human misery, God is present in the most indigent of circumstances, God is compassionate and gracious, and God forgives those whom we struggle to forgive. God abides with the "least of these" with a lavishly extravagant love and broad banqueting table.

Kingdom of God

A few of the missionaries mentioned a broader understanding of the kingdom of God—leading me to think that the "kingdom of God" is a phrase commonly discussed/read in WMF culture and/or its usage may reflect WMF staffers' tendency to come from an evangelical heritage. The staffers mentioned that their conception what the kingdom of God is had broadened due to service with WMF.

> Since moving to Argentina, I've been challenged and stretched in listening and in understanding spiritualities in different cultural contexts. My perspective on the church and the kingdom of God has broadened through readings and discussions. My concept of the kingdom of God has expanded a great deal—I was more narrow-minded before WMF.
>
> My understanding of the kingdom of God has matured through WMF. I see God's desire to make ALL things new.

Staffers felt that God included many more people in his kingdom than they thought, including those whom they would have previously judged as unworthy. Due to their time with WMF, interviewees realized that the boundaries of God's kingdom are much more expansive than they had thought.

How We've Changed: Reflections on New Habits

For WMF staffers, change in the way they cared for themselves and their health came both because of life experience on the field, and through the new initiatives of Community Care.[16] The senior staff who had been in the mission field for a decade or more had learned that they had to live sustainably, or they wouldn't make it in their challenging settings. I divide the habits into personal and institutional because not only have WMF individuals made concrete changes in the way they live, but also the WMF corporate culture has shifted to greater health.

Personal Changes in Habits: Spiritual Practices

More than any other habit, missionaries mentioned spiritual practices that were taught and encouraged through WMF and its Community Care as being life-giving. WMF's emphasis on the active contemplative life and promotion of practices such as centering prayer, spiritual direction, and

---

16. I focus here mainly on changes in habits that came as a result of Community Care. One factor mentioned by several female missionaries, which had nothing to do with Community Care, was pregnancy/having children. People felt that they made better choices for their own health because they now had children on the field with them. One staffer said, "Having children forces us into good rhythms and health. There is always the tension of wanting to do more, but we decided to limit our nights out (meeting with street children). We do need to be at home; we choose more prudently (how we work) because of children."

PART TWO—Habits of Health in Christian Community

personal retreat offered staffers new habits that sustained them in their work with impoverished women and children. Several staffers active abroad gave testimony to how WMF's emphasis on spiritual practices has impacted their own lives.

> As WMF began exploring contemplative practices it became life-giving. The emphasis on spiritual formation and covenant, on centering prayer and getting together as a community . . . WMF offers lots more resources and tools for incorporating spiritual rhythms into life—both for our personal and corporate journey.

> The emphasis on prayer practices and contemplative activism has been a blessing. It's the only way I've been able to continue—by keeping the emphasis on Christ and letting my actions flow out of that relationship.

Other staffers spoke more specifically about new habits in their lives as a result of WMF's emphasis on contemplative spirituality. Several mentioned the importance spiritual direction now plays for them.

> Spiritual direction has been real life-changing. Someone leading me . . . who has encouraged and supported me personally (has been significant) . . . it shapes how I know God.

> I have a spiritual director through Community Care. I feel loved and welcomed as I am, I feel loved and invited to take care of myself and to be the best of who I am.

Others spoke of the significance of sabbatical and personal retreats for enhancing their health.

> Every three months I take a retreat—I'm more intentional now about getting away with a plan to be alone. In my eighth year of service I took a sabbatical. I did a pilgrimage in Italy and spent time in a New Hampshire farmhouse—in my own space but also close enough to be near family for three months. I enjoyed nature, I took an art class. I spent the last part of it doing a family heritage discovery trip . . . the sabbatical was excellent. Three months of being still was rejuvenating.

> I take personal retreats. I will be going on sabbatical next year; the preparation for sabbatical has been good. In Calcutta we have developed practices out of community care, like getting out of the city every three months. We need a place of rest and

> relief—just something to give us a break. The retreats are born out of an invitation to take care of ourselves. Each community forms its own way...

The contemplative practices supported and advocated by Community Care has shaped people into new spiritual habits that they find life-affirming and that renders them more whole.

Personal Changes in Habits: Healthy Rhythms and Sustainability

More than any other words, I heard "rhythm of life" and "sustainability" mentioned by the staffers to describe how their lives are now different through Community Care. By "rhythm" they meant a regular pattern of spiritual practices incorporated into their labor. By "sustainability" they pointed toward a way of life in which they can maintain their physical, emotional, and physical health—and a long-term commitment to the mission field—in the midst of extraordinarily trying living conditions. Missionaries described ways in which they were learning both to live in a healthy rhythm and sustainably.

> We were aware of the challenges in starting a new field. We know the times of running ragged. We've had lots of conversations about sustainability ... we are trying to make good rhythms for ourselves, of being more aware in order to take retreats, of physically stepping away from the city. We finally joined a gym ... we made Wednesdays a day of spiritual and emotional development—a day of prayer...

> I am learning that my stability and ability to stay on the field is integrally interwoven with physical wellbeing. When I let that go everything else goes out of wack. I am learning disciplines in all areas of life, I am choosing to exercise. All disciplines feed into everything else. I choose these things so that I can be sustainable...

> I try to live in a rhythm of life and in communion with God, with life in community and life in mission. My personal rhythm is divided into that. I try to be intentional about how I'm giving necessary priority.

> In Community Care we try to emphasize boundaries for staff ... I'm realizing the space that I need for introverted time. I try

PART TWO—Habits of Health in Christian Community

> to model a 8:30am–4:30pm work day and not be at the office longer than that. We encourage each other to stay in the 40 hour work week, but also to have the space to say that I need some time. We have the freedom to do that—to have healthy rhythms in life and work by not working a ton and taking a break, but establishing rhythms.

Personal Changes in Habits: Better Physical Health

Not surprisingly, out of their experiences with Community Care missionaries described better personal physical health and practices—much like the United Methodist clergy had better diet and exercise habits after CHI's intervention.

> I am now eating better and making exercise a priority. I'm taking more time for relationships. I am slowing down to be incarnational.

> I've started to value a healthy diet; I wasn't as motivated before. I value exercise, I've learned to say "no" to things on the weekend. I practice the spirituality of living the Sabbath; I have a long, slow meal with friends on that day.

> I'm more accepting in attending to my own health and accepting my own limitations. I hit the gym three times a week . . . I'm more aware of how to eat and how creation is tied in. Sleep is always a challenge but with activity and food I sleep better . . .

For WMF staffers, greater attention to diet and exercise flowed out of prior commitments to a spiritual life and to a wholesome rhythm. By nurturing their spirits, they became more aware of the need to nurture and care for their bodies. Aquinas's holistic anthropology confirms such findings; the inextricability of body and soul indicates that improvements in the spiritual life has repercussions into the physical, and vice versa.

Institutional Changes for Healthier Habits: Supportive Community

WMF emphasizes community throughout its organization; community is one their lifestyle celebrations. On the international fields, missionaries live and work together in community, both with other American staffers and with the people of that nation. The WMF staffers affirmed that the

Word Made Flesh

institution really practices community in regards to health and wellbeing. WMF gives the missionaries a strong sense of belonging and a group where they feel understood and appreciated. This practice of community was there before the installment of Community Care, but seems to have been enhanced and made even more intentional with the establishment of this program. A few of the missionaries' testimonies:

> WMF values community and I feel I am in a safe place. I know that I will be cared for and valued. Community is a lifestyle celebration and it is in WMF ethics and in relationships between individuals—and in settings like this (the Gathering) every three years.

> I was emotionally exhausted... WMF supported me and helped me find a counselor. I have a spiritual director through community care. I feel loved and welcomed with who I am (by WMF staff). I feel loved and invited to take care of myself, to be the best of who I am.

> It helps to be part of a larger community that values health ... the emphasis on (well-being) as a community is celebrated rather than criticized.

Institutional Changes for Healthier Habits: Greater Resources

Through Community Care WMF has developed a practice of equipping missionaries with resources to live well. From books and spiritual director referrals to a sabbatical guide and practice, WMF now provides tangible ways to support its staff in living a whole life.

> WMF is introducing new books and resources that could help us all. It (WMF) has begun to integrate more preparation reading (for missionaries entering field) ...

> We've developed a three year process for formation, with the emphasis in the first year on spiritual formation with limited named responsibilities; years 2 and 3 focus on rhythm of life—new staff are partnered with a senior staff. These years focus on vocational discernment tied together with formation ... we've also added resources on mental and emotional health with different tools and testing. We have tools for physical health and contacts and references for spiritual directors.

PART TWO—Habits of Health in Christian Community

This wealth of resources simply wasn't present or available to staff before the creation of Community Care; through these resources staff have become much healthier individuals and communities of service.

Institutional Changes for Healthier Habits: Openness to Transformation

The senior staff described WMF as an organization that has truly undergone a transformation in the area of wellness. From a culture of "sink or swim" prior to 2004, by 2010 it had become a community in which new staffers felt that their health was valuable and deserving of care. Long-time staffers made these observations about WMF's practice of transformation:

> The community care center has put options in place for the community. Before there was a lack of initiative in receiving resources as gift; people tended to be against relationship tools, retreat policies. They didn't want to be told what to do, and when told to do it they pushed back. (Staffers) didn't receive well . . . there was some guilt in receiving the gift of caring for self—it sounds like a luxury. Now we've moved from feeling bad to receiving limitations and needs as graces . . . This allows us to be accepting of others' needs and limitations . . .

> We've come a long way in this area (wellbeing/health). At every point where a need was brought up then Community Care tries to meet that need, from sabbatical to connecting us with spiritual directors . . .

> We are learning from others that have gone before about sustainability and simplicity. There is an emphasis on incarnational ministry. There is always a tension between life in the States and life in the field that can create stress. Others before us tried to live as Sierra Lionians. They burned out and left the field quicker. They didn't have good hygiene or electricity. Now we are really on the side of sustainability. We set our budgets higher, we cook for ourselves, we spend money on the internet. Finding comforts that feel like home can help in the long term—running at a deficit doesn't allow for long term service and being emotionally and spiritually healthy.

As a result of the institution of Community Care, WMF now embodies greater care and attention to matters of health than prior to its presence. As an organization WMF made a seismic change in its attention toward and consciousness of wellbeing—and it continues to be committed to growing in its support of health.

Discussion of Results

A Firmer Theological Foundation on Health/Body

WMF, as an organization without any seminary-trained theologians, is making a commendable effort to train and catechize its staff through a new formation program. Those going into the mission field are required to read a wide array of books/articles in missiology, spirituality, theology, and community care (which includes books on self-care in the mission field, WMF Community Care publications, counseling/therapy, etc.). In effect WMF is creating a contextual mini-seminary program for its staff in order to prepare them for the rigors that await them in the field.

However, WMF could benefit from more specific attention to theology of the body. Given the either strongly detrimental or absent teachings on the body that the staffers receive from their churches of origin, the community commences their WMF service with significant hindrances to seeing their bodies as worthy of care. Such damaging embedded theology results in denial of ones own needs (martyrdom/sacrifice), excessive work, disregard of exercise/diet/sleep, and refusal to seek out assistance (through counseling, spiritual direction, etc) from others—traits that have all been displayed by WMF staff members.

In order to correct and rehabilitate damaging theologies of the body from childhood/adolescence, WMF could require additional theological reading, as well as promote open discussion among staff members of their experiences relating to the body/health in their childhoods/adolescences.[17] A robust catechesis that affirms the body as good could be life-giving to current and future missionaries who have had a dearth of such teaching.

---

17. Some possibilities for reading might include: Paulsell, *Honoring the Body*; Griffith, *Born Again Bodies*; and Swinton, *Raging with Compassion*.

PART TWO—Habits of Health in Christian Community

The Theology of Aquinas on Health and Habit

In addition to a stronger theology of the body, WMF could benefit from reflection upon Aquinas's virtue theology. Aquinas offers to this organization a theological grounding for the practices housed within Community Care. Thomas's understanding of the practice of healthcare as leading to lives of flourishing with deeper relationships with God and neighbor affirms WMF staffers' experiences, while at the same providing Christian language around the WMF commitments to holistic healthcare. Like for the United Methodist clergy, Aquinas's understanding of habits as directing people to a life of greater virtue and love offers the invaluable insight for missionaries that the care of oneself is worth it. Aquinas's theology of habit offers a hermeneutic to describe how WMF was able to change from a culture of sink or swim to one of flourishing, and provides a helpful foundation for further change within the organization.

Virtues

Many of the interviewees articulated that they were changed persons because of participation in Community Care's programs; they have richer relationships with God, better physical health, and more attention to holistic rhythms in their days. They've relaxed their workaholism and now cultivate deeper relationships with the people in their communities. Without being trained in the cardinal virtues the staffers nonetheless demonstrated that they had become more virtuous people.

Prudence emerged as a virtue most practiced by the missionaries. They have learned to say "yes" to the care of their health, and "no" to choices that would entrench them in abuse of their body. They choose to go on personal retreats, to take sabbatical, and to employ contemplative prayer practices daily. As Aquinas says, they have learned the rightness of appetite so that they know choose rightly the good.[18]

Through life on the field and through Community Care the staffers also learned to practice temperance. They mitigated their addiction to work, they exercised more, and they prepared better meals. Interviewees also choose to engage in disciplines that supported their attempts to live in the mean of good health, such as spiritual direction or joining a gym.

---

18. Aquinas, *ST* I-II 51.4.

WMF employees seemed deeply aware of the injustices in their communities that prevented their, and the local inhabitants, cultivation of health. Unsafe streets, lack of exercise facilities/gyms, and lack of access to adequate food/safe water all factor into unhealthy lifestyles in their communities. Community Care's focus seems now to be primarily upon the care of staffers' health; future growth in the institution could focus upon bettering the health of the communities in which the staffers serve.

Lastly, the missionaries who first adopted strategies to care for their health when WMF's culture was that of "sink or swim" demonstrated courage. The first person to join a gym in Peru and the first staffer to seek spiritual direction made the first brave steps toward changing WMF toward the care of health and wellbeing. Even now, with a supportive culture, missionaries must remain stalwart and committed to the care of their health in other cultural contexts, in which few locals have the resources or knowledge to tend to their bodies.

Further Areas for WMF to Address

WMF could definitely benefit from more pastoral care and leadership toward its staff. Secondly, WMF might gain from examining the administrative burden placed upon senior staff members. Thirdly, WMF could work on clarifying the mission and offerings of Community Care for staff in the field. Fourthly, WMF could profit from continuing to learn from their experienced missionaries about habits of health. In particular, women who had families while in service had learned a great deal about how to live sustainably for long-term mission field service.

Conclusion to WMF Results

The experience of the missionaries with Community Care indicates that intentionality around health/wellbeing changes people's experience of life and work as a whole. Regrettably, due to the timing of these interviews toward the beginning of my research, I didn't ask the WMF staffers to reflect specifically upon Aquinas's theology of habit. However, they embodied Thomas's teaching that those disciplines we practice daily shape us into more virtuous people. As a result of new practices ranging from contemplative prayer to home-cooked meals the missionaries lead changed lives. Compared to the era prior to Community Care's inception, the staff

PART TWO—Habits of Health in Christian Community

live with greater vitality and passion. Their relationships with God broadened and so too did their relationships with other human beings in their community. The WMF staff lived into *eudaimonia*. From new habits of health they entered into true flourishing. I'll close this section with one missionary's observation about how she has changed during her course of time with WMF:

> I've seen people not make it because they aren't taking care of themselves. I've seen people needing to leave, wearing themselves out. We've [Word Made Flesh] learned so much. It parallels my own journey . . . I wanted a healthier way to live life.

Comparisons and Contrasts between CHI and WMF

Both the clergy and missionaries mentioned struggles with workaholism, sacrifical/martyrdom impulses, and time management (always more work to do). Since both groups work in service to others under the name of Christ, the sharing of similar pressures in regards to health/wellbeing comes as no surprise. If anything, missionaries had even more work stressors due to the destitute nature of their surroundings. In and through all of the vocational stressors experienced (in often similar ways) by clergy and missionaries, both found healthier ways of living through new programs (CHI and Commmunity Care, respectively). It is here that similarities end.

WMF Made Institutional Changes, CHI Did Not

A striking difference between the new habits of health in the communities was the level of corporate change within WMF. The individual missionaries spoke of changes in their own lives, but they also described the difference that the creation of Community Care made in the life of their organization. Their language as a whole was much more communal—with more use of the first person plural to describe how changes were made and experienced. Clearly with WMF, the inception of Community Care, which was developed internally, confirmed and solidified a cultural shift within the whole organization to holistic, sustainable lifestyles. Staff felt that not only were they different, but WMF was healthier, too.

Among the United Methodist clergy, the Clergy Health Initiative caused dramatic changes in individuals. However, as an outside organization funded through endowment and grant money, CHI didn't evoke systemic change within the Western/North Carolina Conferences of the United Methodist Church, or the church as a whole. Though CHI has eventual goals of transmitting change throughout the whole institution, the pilot program really only effected measurable change in the lives of individuals. The institution as a whole remained largely the same.

Institutional Support versus Institutional Suspicion

Closely liked to institutional change is the WMF staff's feeling of support for their organization. Missionaries raved about the post-2004 WMF's commitment to their health and wellbeing, to contemplative practices, and to sabbatical/retreat. Several testified to ways in which WMF's offering of leaves of absence or counseling/spiritual direction was life-giving to them. The staff painted a picture of supportive relationships and resources that sustained their health.

In contrast, most United Methodist clergy felt a complete lack of support from their leadership and conferences. They felt suspicious of sharing any weakness or illness for fear of it compromising their ability to advance in church appointments. No one offered any testimonies of support that they had received from district superintendents or bishops. Instead, the clergy described an atmosphere of fear and suspicion within the organization that inhibited their own individual efforts to live a life of flourishing. Several also despaired for the fates of vibrant, young, hopeful clergy who enter into ministry and then get life crushed out of them through miserable appointments.

Youthfulness versus Age

Word Made Flesh is just over twenty years old, and maintains a dynamic ability to change and adapt. It evolved the Community Care program fairly quickly with the support, endorsement, and labor of missionaries already on the field. Its light-footed ability to transform itself testifies both to the youthfulness of the leadership (all of the interviewees were under age 45), and to the smaller size of the institution—with only 200 staff. However, WMF does appear to be gaining some baggage of institutionalism as it ages, with increasing burdens of administration upon its senior staff.

The United Methodist Church, on the other hand, has tens of thousands of clergy, eight million members, and a few centuries of age. Both the size and the age of the institution inhibit systemic change; even the clergy have more age than a WMF staffer—all of the clergy I interviewed were over the age of 42. CHI wisely chose to begin its program of wellness by focusing on under 100 clergy in small geographic areas within North Carolina. Systemic change toward wellness in a system which currently does little to encourage clergy health will be a process years, perhaps even decades in the making.

Theological Training

None of the WMF staff had a Master of Divinity or an equivalent. All of the theological training in the organization came through independent reading and discussions, or now through the new formation program. In contrast, the clergy all had either a Master of Divinity or had trained under the Course of Study for local pastors. The clergy could clearly articulate theologies of the body and theological reasons for the care of health, whereas the WMF staff lacked such catechesis. Even with such training, the clergy struggled just as much as the missionaries in caring for their health. Whether the theology articulated was academic or practical, both groups of service professionals needed outside support, whether it be CHI or Community Care, to support and encourage them into new ways of being.

Coherence versus Confusion

The CHI, run by a staff of dedicated professionals (many of whom were not United Methodists themselves), is a clearly organized program. All of the participants knew what was required of them, and could easily describe what the program offered to them. By contrast, the Community Care of Word Made Flesh seemed more haphazard and still in formation. Many of the participants couldn't clearly articulate what it was. Several of them described benefits in their spiritual life that came more from inherent aspects of WMF rather than from any intervention of Community Care. As Community Care ages and becomes more intrinsic to the organization, one could expect to see better organization and clearer understandings of its services among WMF staffers.

Conclusion

Both CHI and WMF evidenced that the Thomist practice of good habits of health transforms lives. The clergy and missionaries became more lovely and more virtuous, both as individuals and as members of their ecclesial communities. Through the work of CHI and Community Care the interviewees developed greater holistic health, which encompassed their minds, bodies, and spirits. They ate better, exercised more, prayed deeper, retreated more frequently, and complained less. They became more virtuous—more prudent, temperate, courageous, and just. They fell deeper in love with God and they had richer relationships with other human beings as a result of their commitments to new habits of health. As they oriented their lives to the *telos* of God through caring for their wellbeing, the interviewees experienced greater flourishing. They became more like the love of God as they became healthier—just as Aquinas taught centuries ago.

Thus, both groups could benefit enormously from intentional study of the theology of Thomas Aquinas. Aquinas offers a substantive theological support for the work of Community Care and CHI, and gives a rich hermeneutic to the commitments of both of these groups to health. Where the groups struggle to be healthy, both individually and corporately, Aquinas offers further recommendations for greater habituation. For example, in a Methodist church that struggles with an antiquated appointment system, Aquinas gestures to the virtue of courage and the significance of an ecclesial body striving toward God, rather than *teloi* of power or prestige.

Even without the benefits of study of Aquinas and with the acknowledgement of vicious habits within their systems, The United Methodist clergy and the WMF missionaries demonstrate the validity of habits of health. They embodied Karl Barth's teaching that "we must do whatever we can to be healthy and faithful."[19] Their healthy habits helped them to nurture the transformation that God's love began and will complete.[20] Their new practices guided them, and guide them still, into God's graced promises for happiness and true flourishing.

---

19. Barth, *Doctrine of Creation*, 359.
20. Wadell, *Primacy of Love*, 109.

11

Conclusion: Habits of Health and the Church

Habits of Health

AQUINAS'S ADAPTATION OF ARISTOTELIAN HABIT OFFERS A MORAL STRATegy in which the nurture of habits that sustain good health constitute part of the virtuous life with God. Aquinas's understanding of habit as fully embodied/ensouled and inclusive of the passions empowers Christians with the agency necessary to care for their own health. By mobilizing the will and reason people initiate habits of health that, when practiced faithfully, lead them to greater prudence, temperance, justice, and courage. As Christians continue living into habits of health, their virtuous lives guide them deeper into love with God, and with their neighbor.

Such virtuous lives require continuous vigilance, dedication and intentionality. In the disease-rampant American context, health requires a virtuous effort—an effort beautifully described in Aquinas's account of habit. A couple of Christian groups have courageously incorporated strategies that embody Thomistic habits—their efforts at health have indeed changed them into healthier, more virtuous people. Not only are blood pressures lower and eating habits better among Clergy Health Initiative (CHI) participants and Word Made Flesh (WMF) staff, but also they are more loving with parishoners/members of their communities and more vibrant in ministry. By living into the virtue-based medicine provided through CHI and WMF's Community Care, many participants have been transformed.

Paul Wadell describes this transformation well as he writes,

> Habits provide the transition necessary for genuine humanity, the link between who we are at any moment of our lives and who

we must become if we are not to fall short of our promise. How do we become the most we can become? Through a lifetime of virtuous behavior. And the reason is that the virtues perfect us by forming us in the goodness of our grandest possibility.[1]

Through the modifications of habits of health CHI participants, WMF staff, and all the rest of us can become new, grander persons. We can become more lovely and holy. As we transform to become more like the love of God, we live into habit's true ends. Sustained by the Holy Spirit, we are able to embody *eudaimonia*. Habits of health perfected in God's grace promise healing, wholeness, happiness, and peace so that we are able to love as we have been loved. Through habits of health sustained by charity we become beloved friends of God and our neighbors. Through habits of health we—and the creation and creatures around us--truly flourish.

The Church

Exactly this communal orientation of habits of health distinguishes Aquinas's moral strategy; our individual practices enable us to serve others with greater Christian love. We cultivate health not only to be more like the people God created us to be, but also because health constitutes a Christian obligation. By the care of our own health, we are better able to care for the health of others and for the health of our ecclesial communities. Health, then, becomes a witness of Christian faith and love.

Indeed, the practice of the cardinal virtues requires more than one person; for example, in order to be just we must have a neighbor with whom we can share God's largesse to us. We cannot live morally without one another. Just as our very bodies depend upon the sustenance, work, and nurture of other bodies, so too is our healthy moral action interdependent upon another.

Therefore, our practices of habits of health aren't something we do on our own as highly motivated individuals, but as people formed by and cared for by others.[2] For Aquinas we are not just individuals cultivating health toward the love of God; habits of health are an inescapably communal endeavor. As followers of Christ, our practices of care for

1. Wadell, *Primacy of Love*, 115.
2. The communal aspect of practices of health distinguishes "habit" from a multitude of self-improvement/weight-loss/fitness programs on the market, which focus solely on individual betterment and enhancement.

Conclusion: Habits of Health and the Church

our bodies are inextricably interwoven with the care of other, vulnerable bodies around us and with the care of the creation that sustains our lives. Wendell Berry encompasses such ideas when he writes, "community is in the fullest sense a place and all its creatures—it is the smallest unit of health and to speak of the health of an isolated individual is a contradiction in terms."[3]

Aquinas, following Aristotle, used the term "friendship" to describe how our bodies are interrelated to one another through the practice of virtuous habits and the pursuit of the good.[4] In his discussion of charity in the *Secundae Secundae* he writes that our human friendships are based upon our communion with God and that true happiness requires such relationships. Aquinas sees the circle of friendship ever widening so that as we love our friends and wish them good we come to love their friends, thus participating in an ecclesial community of love that is connected to one another through the love of Christ.[5] These friendships then sustain and encourage us in the practice of habits of health.

Yet, even more than eating apples together, friends care for one another when the apples still fail to prevent cancer. Friends in Christ support one another when health diminishes and finitude presents itself. Joel Shuman states "in this sense the first step of acquiring virtue is in fact, as both Aristotle and Aquinas suggest, a matter of taking time to act virtuous."[6] Friends take time for one another by practicing habits that sustain a vision of healing in the midst of brokenness. Friends in Christ are truly the best kind to have, because not only do they help us to be more virtuous people, but they enable us to endure suffering in life by orienting us to deeper friendship with God. Our life together as friends, as bodies who are linked together, is sustained by the body of Christ (the church) and the body of Christ as shared in the Eucharistic table and a

---

3. Berry, "Health is Membership," in *Another Turn of the Crank*, 90. A practice that cares for creation and for people is church participation in Community Sustained Agriculture (CSA), in which a congregation supports a farmer, and in turn feasts upon fresh local produce. Such practices flow from the inner commitments of the church community, and become habits of health that benefit everyone, including the land. Many churches are growing community gardens, nourishing themselves and their neighborhood with fresh produce—another example of a communal health habit.

4. Aristotle writes that "perfect friendship is the friendship of men who are good, and alike in virtue; for these wish well alike to each other *qua* good, and they are good in themselves. Aristotle, *Nicomachean Ethics* 8:3 1156.

5. Aquinas, *ST* II-IIae.23.1 in Bauerschmidt, *Holy Teaching*, 154–55.

6. Shuman, *Body of Compassion*, 146.

PART TWO—Habits of Health in Christian Community

life of liturgy.[7] Wendell Berry writes that "when we say the word "body" theologically, we cannot distinguish in an absolute way whether we mean our own human bodies, Jesus's human body, Christ's bodily presence in the elements of the Eucharist, or the social body called the church."[8] Thus, everybody becomes more whole through the practices of habits of health.

Therefore, in response to the query, "what is health for" one could answer not only for a virtuous life, but also that health is for everyone else. Habits of health order us to charity for others. Our practices of health enable us to love others more deeply and to serve our neighbors, our church, and our creation.

A Hope for Charity

My whole motivation for this exploration of habit came out of my journey of learning how to tend to my health in the midst of chronic illness. I wanted to learn how to understand my efforts as somehow holding the potential for virtue. I yearned to learn how in and through increasing disability I could yet love God, and love others.

I've now had over a decade of experience at being a chronically ill Christian. I take a huge handful of vitamins without consciously thinking about it (on my good days)—and none of them remotely resemble the taste of gummy candy. When my legs no longer could run (and oh, how I had loved to run!), I cultivated cycling and an abiding practice of yoga. I learned how I could endure physical pain and continue to live days filled with goodness.

I failed miserably, though, at how to live sustainably and in a healthy rhythm in service to the Christian community. When my first "attack" hit, I was working as an associate pastor in a large suburban church. I was almost burned out, and I had barely begun my career in ministry. Though I loved that community deeply, I knew that I had practiced the "24/7" mentality described by so many clergy in the Clergy Health Initiative. I was literally on the path of making a martyr out of myself. Others more skilled than I—others like the clergy and missionaries whom

---

7. Bell, *Ritual Theory, Ritual Practce*, 96, as used in Shuman, *Body of Compassion*, 124. In the liturgy the formation of individual bodies is caught up in the grand drama of ritual and embodied practices that shapes the whole community. The liturgy shapes us into friendship with God and for one another so that we live lives of wholeness and health.

8. Berry, "Health Is Membership," in *Another Turn of the Crank*, 90–91.

Conclusion: Habits of Health and the Church

I studied—could initiate and practice virtuous habits while in the same service setting. However, I needed to leave to learn more how to live toward flourishing.

I went back to school and surrounded myself with the wisdom of the Christian community. I found friends who taught me about how to live a wholesome life toward God—or rather, these friends found me. Thomas Aquinas, whom I'm sure could have never conceived of a Protestant clergywoman, nonetheless took me by the hand, and gave me the gift of *Prima Secundae* questions forty-nine to fifty-two. This work has really been an effort at a close reading of those questions, and their insights for health in the Christian community.

I found other, unlikely friends, too. John Wesley shared with me about the significance of health practices for the people called Methodists. Pope John Paul II lent me great wisdom about sharing in our sufferings with Christ, while Karl Barth urged me onward that my effort to be healthy toward God is indeed faithful. Mystics such as Hadewijch, Margorie Kempe, and Angela of Foligno showed me the beauty of lives caught up in love of God. Even more importantly, a historically African American United Methodist Church took me in as a daughter, and showed me how people have lived with suffering for centuries—and how to praise God through that pain. They even let me sing about it in their gospel choir, for which I'm forever grateful.

In short, I received great charity from the Christian community—both those who spoke to me through written words, and those who hugged and prayed for me. I was loved into a deeper friendship with God through the incarnate, corporate body of Christ. I received great healing, even though my actual illness didn't improve.

After my time of being held by the church and learning about habits of health, I went back into serving the church. This time, I had a tiny rural church with a small membership. I no longer worked 24/7. I loved that dear people with the love of God, which meant I also took care of myself. I let my sermons be prepared as much by prayer as by work. Together, we really flourished.

Now, I, with a still limping leg and generally poor balance, offer this writing up to you. For my fellow servants in Christ, clergy and missionaries, I pray that it might assist you in cultivating healthy habits. I pray that this work might in some tiny measure preserve you from my mistakes, and that the courageous clergy in CHI and missionaries in Word Made Flesh might inspire you. I pray that in some small way, this

PART TWO—Habits of Health in Christian Community

writing, which came from the charity expressed to me by the Christian community, might be an act of charity to you. May you live deeply into habits of health—and find in the end the happiness of God's love. May you flourish.

Appendix

Interview Questions

Interview Questions for Staff Members of Word Made Flesh

(All interviews will take place during the annual Staff Gathering at Lied Lodge, July 15–22.)

1. Describe how you became employed with Word Made Flesh.
2. Describe the nature of your work with WMF.
3. What impact does your work have upon your overall health and wellbeing?
4. Describe your knowledge of and participation in the wellness programs of WMF.
5. How has your participation in sabbatical or other wellness programs of WMF affected your health?
6. What have you learned about yourself, your body, and other people's bodies/health through your participation in WMF's wellness program?
7. How has your participation in WMF's program on wellness impacted how you make daily decisions about health and wellbeing? Has your behavior changed?
8. Do you feel you make more prudent decisions about your health as a result of participation in WMF's wellness program?

Appendix

9. How has your relationship to God and to other people changed as a result of participation in WMF's wellness programs?

Interview Questions for Clergy Participants in Clergy Health Initiative

(All interviews took place in North Carolina, January 3–5, 2011.)
State number of years in ministry, number of appointments, seminary, describe current church setting

1. How were you shaped in your childhood and adolescence to think about the care of your body and health—both through your homelife and in the church?

2. Now as an adult and actively serving clergyperson, how would you describe your theological understanding of the body and of practices directed to caring for your health?

3. Are there any scriptures that guide your understanding of the care for health?

4. What may hinder you or other clergy from cultivating habits to care for your health? What may be theological hindrances?

5. In thinking on ways for clergy to care for their health, I have often thought that John Wesley offers helpful theology and practice. I'd like to briefly share about Wesley and health now (you may know some of this already) and then get your reaction to how this might motivate you to do the difficult work of caring for yourself. First, Wesley wrote the Primitive Physic, a bestseller in his day, of home remedies so that people could care for themselves without incurring high physician or drug costs. He started a free apothecary in London for those who couldn't afford medicine. However, most of all, he strongly advocated in numerous writings for the importance of preventative self-care—for adequate hygiene and sleep, for exercise and a local diet—as a significant part of ones life of faith. Theologically, John Wesley understood practices of health and healing as fruits of the journey of sanctification; they were acts of goodness and love for God and for one another.[1] How might any of this (meaning Wesley's own com-

---

1. Holifield, *Health and Medicine*, 22. "Wesley's interest in health and medicine reflected his concern about the salvation of souls . . . [Christians] cared for the body because they cared for the soul." On the journey of sanctification, Christians cared for the sick because it was the loving thing to do. For a more in-depth discussion of

mitment to practices of healthcare, both personal and communal) help you in your own practices of health and that of your church?

6. In my own thinking about ways for clergy and Christians to nurture their health, I have reflected that the theology of St. Thomas Aquinas offers us resources. I'd like to share now about Aquinas on health, and then get your reaction as to how this might be helpful for your own health practices. Aquinas argues in questions 49–54 of the Prima Secundae in the *Summa Theologiae* that the nurture of good habits leads to a life of virtue, and ultimately, flourishing with God. I have a hypothesis that the understanding of habits as virtuous offers a greater end (*telos*) to our own personal care of our health. In this theology my care of my own health becomes much more than just an improvement of my weight or blood pressure; such healthcare, when directed toward God, becomes a way for me to love God and my neighbor more deeply. For Aquinas care of personal health isn't selfish or narcissistic; rather, healthcare comprises good habits that make us more virtuous and lead us into deeper relationship with God.

What, if any of this, would be helpful for you taking care of your own health?

1. What have you learned about yourself, your body, and your health through your participation in the Clergy Health Initiative's (CHI) pilot program?
2. What, if any, changes have you made in your daily decisions and behavior concerning your health and wellbeing?
3. What advice would you now offer to a clergy colleague who is struggling with health issues?
4. What changes, if any, have you experienced in your relationships with God and to other people as a result of your participation in CHI's wellness programs?

Wesley's commitment to preventative care through diet, exercise, sleep, and the cold regime, see Randy Maddox's essay "Wesley on Holistic Health and Healing."

Bibliography

Aquinas, Thomas. *De Anima Quaestio disputata de Anima*. Edited by J. H. Robb. Toronto: Pontifical Institute of Mediaeval Studies, 1968.
———. *Summa Theologiae*. Vol. 22, *Dispositions for Human Acts*. Translated by Anthony Kenny. Cambridge: Cambridge University Press, 1964
———. *Summa Theologiae*. Vol. 23, *Virtue*. Translated by W. D. Hughes. Cambridge: Cambridge University Press, 1969.
———. *Treatise on Happiness*. Translated by John A. Oesterle. Notre Dame: University of Notre Dame Press, 1983.
———. *Treatise on the Virtues*. Translated by John A. Oesterle. Notre Dame: University of Notre Dame Press, 1984.
Aristotle. *Categories*. In *The Basic Works of Aristotle*. Edited by Richard McKeon. New York: Random House, 1941.
———. *Eudemian Ethics*. In *Aristotle: Athenian Constitution, Eudemian Ethics, Virtues and Vices*. Translated by H. Rackham. Loeb Classical Library. Cambridge, MA: Harvard University Press, 1980.
———. *Metaphysics*. In *The Basic Works of Aristotle*. Edited by Richard McKeon. New York: Random House, 1941.
———. *Nicomachean Ethics*. Translated by Terence Irwin. Cambridge: Cambridge University Press, 2000.
Barth, Karl. *The Doctrine of Creation*. Edited by G. Bromiley and T. Torrance. Vol. 3, part 4 of *The Church Dogmatics*. Edinburg: T. & T. Clark, 1961.
Bauerschmidt, Frederick Christian. *Holy Teaching: Introducing the Summa Theologiae of St. Thomas Aquinas*. Grand Rapids: Brazos, 2005.
Berry, Wendell. *Another Turn of the Crank*. Berkeley: Counterpoint, 1995.
Brown, Stephen F. "The Theological Virtue of Faith: An Invitation to an Ecclesial Life of Truth (IIa IIae, qq. 1–16." In *The Ethics of Aquinas*, edited by Stephen Pope, 221–31. Washington, DC: Georgetown University Press, 2002.
Brumberg, Joan Jacobs. *The Body Project: An Intimate History of American Girls*. New York: Vintage, 1998.
Cates, Diana Fritz. *Choosing to Feel: Virtue, Friendship, and Compassion for Friends*. Notre Dame: University of Notre Dame Press, 1997.
Charmaz, K. "Grounded Theory." In *Contemporary Field Research*, edited R. M. Emerson, 335–52. Long Grove, IL: Waveland, 2001.
Clergy Health Initiative. "Clergy Health Initiative." Duke Divinity School. http://divinity.duke.edu/initiatives-centers/clergy-health-initiative.
———. "Spirited Life." Duke Divinity School. http://spiritedlife.org.
Conrad, Peter. "Wellness as Virtue: Morality and the Pursuit of Health." *Culture, Medicine, and Psychiatry* 18 (1994) 385–401.
Curless, Melanie, Tara Haley, and Phileena Heuertz, eds. "Health Guide: A Holistic Approach to Healthy Living." Unpublished document for Word Made Flesh.

Bibliography

Davies, Brian. *The Thought of Thomas Aquinas*. New York: Clarendon, 1992.
Dillon, Dana. "As Soul to Body: The Interior Act of the Will in Thomas Aquinas and the Importance of the First Person Perspective in Accounts of Moral Action." PhD diss., Duke University, 2008.
Dunnington, Kent. "Addiction and Action: Aristotle and Aquinas in Dialogue with Addiction Studies." PhD diss., Texas A&M University, 2007.
———. *Addiction and Virtue: Beyond the Models of Disease and Choice*. Downers Grove, IL: InterVarsity, 2011.
Dwelle, T. L. "Inadequate Basic Preventative Health Measures: Survey of Missionary Children In Sub-Saharan Africa." *Pediatrics* 95 (1995) 733–37.
Eliot, T. S. *The Idea of a Christian Society and Other Writings*. London: Faber & Faber, 1982.
Evans, Abigail Rian. *Redeeming Marketplace Medicine: A Theology of Healthcare*. Cleveland: Pilgrim, 1999.
Ferngren, Gary. *Medicine and Healthcare in Early Christianity*. Baltimore: Johns Hopkins University Press, 2009.
Frei, Hans. *The Eclipse of the Biblical Narrative: A Study in Eighteenth and Nineteenth Century Hermeneutics*. New Haven, CT: Yale University Press, 1974.
Gallagher, David M. "The Will and Its Acts." In *The Ethics of Aquinas*, edited by Stephen Pope, 69–89. Washington, DC: Georgetown University Press, 2002.
Glaser, B. G., and A. L. Strauss. *The Discovery of Grounded Theory: Strategies For Qualitative Research*. Chicago: Aldine, 1967.
Griffith, R. Marie. *Born Again Bodies: Flesh and Spirit in American Christianity*. Berkeley: University of California Press, 2004.
Gunderson, Gary. *Leading Causes of Life*. With Larry Pray. Memphis: Center of Excellence in Faith and Health, Methodist LeBonheur Healthcare, 2006.
Halaas, Gwen Wagstrom. *Ministerial Health and Wellness: 2002 Evangelical Lutheran Church in America*. Chicago: Division for Ministry Board of Pensions, 2002.
Hall, D. E., K. G. Meador, and H. G. Koenig. "Measuring Religiousness in Health Research: Review And Critique." *Journal of Religion and Health* 47 (2008) 134–263.
Hauerwas, Stanley. *Naming the Silences: God, Medicine, and Suffering*. Grand Rapids: Eerdmans, 1990.
Hauerwas, Stanley, and Charles Pinches. *Christians Among the Virtues: Theological Conversations With Ancient and Modern Ethics*. Notre Dame: University of Notre Dame Press, 1997.
Heuertz, Phileena. Interview. February 15, 2010.
———. "Sabbatical Guide: Embracing Creative Absence." Omaha, NE: Word Made Flesh, 2009.
Holifield, E. *Health and Medicine in the Methodist Tradition*. New York: Crossroad, 1986.
Hughes, Melanie Dobson "The Holistic Way: John Wesley's Practical Piety as a Resource for Integrated Healthcare." *Journal of Religion and Health* 47 (2008) 237–52.
Illich, Ivan. *Medical Nemesis: The Expropriation of Health*. New York: Random House, 1976.
Jacobs, Louis. "The Body in Worship." In *Religion and the Body*, edited by Sarah Coakley, 71-89. Cambridge: Cambridge University Press, 1997.

Bibliography

John Paul II. *Letter to the Elderly*. October 1,1999. http://www.vatican.va/holy_father/john_paul_ii/letters/documents/hf_jp-ii_let_01101999_elderly_en.html.

———. *Salvifici Dolores*. February 11, 1984. http://www.vatican.va/holy_father/john_paul_ii/apost_letters/documents/hf_jp-ii_apl_11021984_salvifici-doloris_en.html.

Kant, Immanuel. *Foundations of the Metaphysics of Morals*. Translated by Lewis White Beck. Indianapolis: Bobbs-Merrill, 1969.

Keating, Thomas. *Intimacy with God: An Introduction to Centering Prayer*. New York: Crossroad, 2004.

Kent, Bonnie. "Habits and Virtues." In *Ethics of Aquinas*, edited by Stephen Pope, 116–30. Washington, DC: Georgetown University Press, 2002.

Klima, Gyula. "Man=Body+Soul: Aquinas's Arithmetic of Human Nature." In *Thomas Aquinas: Contemporary Philosophical Perspectives*, edited by Brian Davies, 257–74. Oxford: Oxford University Press, 2002.

Klubertanz, George. *Habits and Virtues: A Philosophical Analysis*. New York: Appleton-Century-Crofts, 1965.

Knight, Kelvin. *Aristotelian Philosophy: Ethics and Politics from Aristotle to MacIntyre*. Cambridge: Polity, 2007.

Lange, W. R., et al. "Missionary Health: The Great Omission." *American Journal of Preventative Medicine* 3 (1987) 332–38.

Lash, Nicholas. *The Beginning and the End of 'Religion.'* Cambridge: Cambridge University Press, 1996.

Lee, C., and J. Iverson-Gilbert. "Demand, Support, and Perception in Family-Related Stress Among Protestant Clergy." *Family Relations* 52 (2003) 249–57.

Levin, Jeffrey. "Religion and Health: Is There an Association, Is It Valid, and Is It Causal?" *Social Science and Medicine* 38 (1994) 1475–82.

Levin, Jeffrey, and Christopher Ellison. "The Religion-Health Connection: Evidence Theory, and Future Directions." *Health Education and Behavior* 25 (1998) 700–20.

Lindner, E. W. *Yearbook of American and Canadian Churches*. Nashville: Abingdon, 2009.

Louth, Andrew. "The Body in Western Christianity." In *Religion and the Body*, edited by Sarah Coakley, 111–30. Cambridge: Cambridge University Press, 1990.

Luther, Martin. *The Freedom of a Christian*. In *Martin Luther's Basic Theological Writings*. Edited by Timothy F. Lull. Minneapolis: Fortress, 2005.

MacIntyre, Alastair. *After Virtue: A Study in Moral Theory*. 2nd ed. Notre Dame: University of Notre Dame Press, 1984.

Maddox, Randy. "John Wesley on Holistic Health and Healing." *Methodist History* 46 (2007) 4–33.

———. *Responsible Grace: John Wesley's Practical Theology*. Nashville: Kingswood, 1994.

Mattison, William. *Introducing Moral Theology: True Happiness and the Virtues*. Grand Rapids: Brazos, 2008.

McKenny, Gerald. "Bioethics, the Body, and the Legacy of Bacon." In *On Moral Medicine*, edited by Stephen Lammers and Allen Verhey, 308–24. 2nd ed. Grand Rapids: Eerdmans, 1998.

———. *To Relieve the Human Condition: Bioethics, Technology, and the Body*. Albany: State University of New York Press, 1997.

Bibliography

Meisenhelder, J. B., and E. N. Chandler. "Frequency of Prayer and Functional Health in Presbyterian Pastors." *Journal for the Scientific Study of Religion* 40 (2001) 323–29.

Milbank, John. *Theology and Social Theory: Beyond Secular Reason*. Oxford: Blackwell, 2006.

Miner, Robert. *Thomas Aquinas on the Passions: A Study of* Summa Theologiae *I-II q. 22-48*. Cambridge: Cambridge University Press, 2009.

Nussbaum, Martha. *The Therapy of Desire: Theory and Practice in Hellenistic Ethics*. Princeton: Princeton University Press, 1994.

Overmyer, Sheryl. "The Wayfarer's Way and Two Guides for the Journey: *The Summa Theologiae* and *Piers Plowman*." PhD diss., Duke University, 2010.

Paulsell, Stephanie. *Honoring the Body: Meditations on a Christian Practice*. San Francisco: Jossey-Bass, 2002.

Pinckaers, Servais-Theodore. "The Sources of the Ethics of St. Thomas Aquinas." In *The Ethics of Aquinas*, edited by Stephen Pope, 17–29. Translated by Mary Thomas Noble. Washington, DC: Georgetown University Press, 2002.

Pope, Stephen. "Overview of the Ethics of Thomas Aquinas." In *The Ethics of Aquinas*, edited by Stephen Pope, 30–56. Washington, DC: Georgetown University Press, 2002.

Porter, Roy. *Flesh in the Age of Reason*. New York: Norton, 2004.

Porterfield, Amanda. *Healing in the History of Christianity*. Oxford: Oxford University Press, 2005.

Prochaska, James, John Norcross, Carlo Diclemente. *Changing for Good: A Revolutionary Six-Stage Program for Overcoming Bad Habits and Moving Your Life Positively Forward*. New York: HarperCollins, 1994.

Proeschold-Bell, Rae Jean, et al. "A Theoretical Model of the Holistic Health of United Methodist Clergy." *Journal of Religion and Health* 50 (April 2009) 700–720. www.springerlink.com/index/k28302144w51x4r5.pdf.

Proeschold-Bell, Rae Jean, and Sara H. LeGrand. "High Rates of Obesity and Chronic Disease Among United Methodist Clergy." *Obesity* 18 (2010) 1867–70.

———. "Physical Health Functioning Among United Methodist Clergy." *Journal of Religion and Health* 51 (2012) 734–42.

Prokes, Mary Timothy. *Toward a Theology of the Body*. Grand Rapids: Eerdmans, 1996.

Risse, Guenter. *Mending Bodies, Saving Souls: A History of Hospitals*. New York: Oxford University Press, 1999.

Rowatt, W. "Stress and Satisfaction in Ministry Families." *Review and Expositor* 98 (2001) 523–43.

Schockenhoff, Eberhard. "The Theological Virtue of Charity (I-IIae, qq.23–46)." In *The Ethics of Thomas Aquinas*, edited by Stephen J. Pope, 244–58. Translated by Grant Kaplan and Frederick Lawrence. Washington, DC: Georgetown University Press, 2002.

Seybold, Klaus, and Ulrich B. Mueller. *Sickness and Healing*. Translated by Douglas W. Stott. Biblical Encounters. Nashville: Abingdon, 1981.

Shuman, Joel James. *The Body of Compassion: Ethics, Medicine, and the Church*. Boulder, CO: Westview, 1999.

Shuman, Joel James, and Keith Meador. *Heal Thyself: Spirituality, Medicine, and the Distortion of Christianity*. Oxford: Oxford University Press, 2003.

Smith, Warren. "Virtue and Theology in Early Christian Ethics." Duke Divinity School Seminar, Durham, NC, January 17, 2008.

Bibliography

Suso, Henry. *The Exemplar with Two German Sermons*. Translated and edited by Frank Tobin. Classics of Western Spirituality. New York: Paulist, 1989.

Taylor, Charles. *Sources of the Self: The Making of the Modern Identity*. Cambridge, MA: Harvard University Press, 1989.

Titus, Craig Steven. *Resilience and the Virtue of Fortitude: Aquinas in Dialogue with the Psychosocial Sciences*. Washington, DC: Catholic University of America Press, 2006.

Torrell, Jean-Pierre. *Aquinas's Summa: Background, Structure, and Reception*. Translated by Benedict M. Guevin. Washington, DC: Catholic University of America Press, 2003.

Turton, D. W., and L. J. Francis. "The Relationship between Attitude toward Prayer and Professional Burnout among Anglican Parochial Clergy in England: Are Praying Clergy Healthier Clergy?" *Mental Health, Religion, and Culture* 10 (2007) 61–74.

University of Virginia Health System. "Hippocrates." Claude Moore Health Sciences. http://www.hsl.virginia.edu/historical/artifacts/antiqua/hippocrates.cfm.

Verhey, Allen. *Reading the Bible in the Strange World of Medicine*. Grand Rapids: Eerdmans, 2003.

Wadell, Paul. *The Primacy of Love: An Introduction to the Ethics of Thomas Aquinas*. Eugene, OR: Wipf & Stock, 1992.

Wesley, John. *Doctrinal Writings: The Appeals to Men of Reason and Religion and Certain Related Open Letters*. Edited by Gerald R. Cragg. Vol. 11 of *The Bicentennial Edition of the Works of John Wesley*, edited by Frank Baker. Nashville: Abingdon, 1975.

———. *Plain Account of the People Called Methodists*, XII, 1–3. Edited by Rupert F. Davies. In *The Methodist Societies I: History, Nature, and Design*, vol. 9 of *The Bicentennial Edition of the Works of John Wesley*, edited by Frank Baker. Nashville: Abingdon, 1989.

———. *The Primitive Physic*. 1791. Reprint, Eugene: Wipf & Stock, 2003.

———. "Thoughts on Nervous Disorders." In *The Works of John Wesley* 11, edited by Thomas Jackson. Grand Rapids: Baker, 1979.

West, Silas. Interview. July 18, 2010.

White, Kevin. "The Passions of the Soul (I-II qq. 22–48)." In *The Ethics of Aquinas*, edited Stephen Pope, 103–15. Washington, DC: Georgetown University Press, 2002.

Winett, R. A., et al. "Guide to Health: Nutrition and Physical Activity Outcomes of a Group Randomized Trial of an Internet-Based Intervention in Churches." *Annals of Behavioral Medicine* 33 (2007) 251–61.

Wirzba, Norman. *The Paradise of God: Renewing Religion in an Ecological Age*. Oxford: Oxford University Press, 2003.

Word Made Flesh. "About WMF." http://www.wordmadeflesh.org/organization/about/.

———. "Formation Materials." Unpublished material, 2010.

World Health Organization. "Preamble to the Constitution of the World Health Organization." www.who.int/about/definition/en/print/html.

———. "World Health Organization Assesses the World's Health Systems." *Theodora.com*. http://www.photius.com/rankings/healthranks.html.

Subject Index

"Accountability" relationships, strengthening of, 93-94
Acquired virtues, 65-71
   Clergy Health Initiative and, 99-100
   courage, 70-71, 99-100, 125
   justice, 68-69, 125
   prudence, 67-68, 99, 124
   relationship to theological virtues, 65n9
   temperance, 69-70, 99, 124
   Word Made Flesh and, 124-25
Action
   as agency of habits of health, 18-19, 32-33
   as habit of health generally, 61-62
Actions of habits of health, 54-63
   action generally, 61-62
   Aquinas on, 54-58
   contemplation, 60-61
   habit and, 57-58
   intellect and, 55n1
   maintenance, 62-63
   overview, 7, 54
   precontemplation, 60
   preparation, 61
   reason and, 56-57
   stages of change, 58-63
   will and, 55-56
Administrative burdens, health and, 111
Ancillary science, 13-14
Angela of Foligno, 135
Aquinas, Thomas (Saint)
   generally, 6-8, 13, 139
   on bodily dispositions, 31n29
   Clergy Health Initiative, philosophy applied to, 78-80, 82, 84, 90-93, 95, 97-99, 101, 129
   on humors, 25n8
   Word Made Flesh, philosophy applied to, 113, 124-25, 129
Aquinas, Thomas (Saint)—on habits of health, 17-38
   actions of habits of health and, 54-58, 60-63
   agency of habit, action as, 18-19, 32-33
   ambivalence of, 41n11
   Aristotle compared, 17-26, 29, 32, 38
   defined, 43nn14-15
   ends of habits of health and, 65-66, 68-69, 72-73
   God as end of habit, 22-23
   grace, habit as infused by, 21-22, 37
   increase, decrease or corruption of habit, 19-21, 33-35
   lasting quality, habit as, 18, 31-32
   overview, 7, 17-18, 24, 38, 131-39
   passion for health and, 47-50, 53
   repetition of habit, 19, 33
   virtue, habit disposing toward, 21, 35-36
Aquinas, Thomas (Saint)—on health, 24-31
   habit, health as, 26-27
   idol, health not deemed, 29
   overview, 24-25, 38
   salvation, health not deemed, 28-29
   status, health as, 25-26
   summum bonum (greatest good), health not deemed, 29

Subject Index

WHO definition of health contrasted, 30–31
Arête (virtue), 14–16
Aristotle
  generally, 7
  holistic approach to health and, 40, 45
  on medicine, 11n14, 14n24, 15n31
Aristotle—on habits of health, 9–16
  actions of habits of health and, 63
  ancillary science, 13–14
  Aquinas compared, 17–26, 29, 32, 38
  ends of habits of health and, 12–16, 68–69
  health as product versus health as practice of virtue, 12–16
  health generally, 11–12
  overview, 6–7, 9, 16, 131, 133
  techne (craft), 13–14
  theoria (rationality), 14–16
  ultimate science, 14–16
  on virtue, 10–11
Augustine (Saint), 18

Barth, Karl, 51–52, 92, 129, 135
Berry, Wendell, 133–34
Body, theology of, 86–89

Cartesian dualism, 39n1, 40–42, 50, 85–86
Catechesis in health, lack of as hindrance to health, 81
Changing for Good: A Revolutionary Six-Stage Program for Overcoming Bad Habits and Moving Your Life Positively Forward (Prochaska, Norcross, and DiClemente), 59
Charity
  impact of habits of health on, 134–36
  as theological virtue, 65–66
Church
  impact of habits of health on, 132–34
  strengthening of through habits of health, 95–97
Clergy Health Initiative, 77–101
  ability to change and adapt, 128
  "accountability" relationships, strengthening of, 93–94
  acquired virtues and, 99–100
  appointment system as hindrance to health, 84–85
  body, theology of, 86–89
  catechesis in health, lack of, 81
  church, strengthening of, 95–97
  coherence in, 128
  confusion in, 128
  constant demand on clergy as hindrance to health, 81–82
  flourishing, increase in, 92–93
  goodness, health and, 88
  "good shepherds," health and, 87
  greater health resulting from new practices, 91–92
  habits of health and, 90–91
  health resources of, 79–80
  hindrances to health, 81–86
  holism and, 89
  institutional changes, lack of, 126–27
  institutional suspicion in, 127
  interview questions, 138–39
  "martyrdom" problem as hindrance to health, 82–83
  new habits adopted by, 91–97
  ongoing journey, habits of health as, 94–95
  overview, 7–8, 78–81, 101, 129
  "people pleaser" problem as hindrance to health, 84
  relationship between theology and health, 97–98
  results of study, 97–101
  "Savior complex" as hindrance to health, 82–83
  stewardship, health and, 87
  study methodology, 80–81
  temple, body as, 88
  theological hindrances to health, 85–86
  theological training in, 128
  time management problem as hindrance to health, 81–82

Subject Index

transformation resulting from habits of health, 131–32
Word Made Flesh compared, 126–28
Community Care. *See* Word Made Flesh
Community Sustained Agriculture (CSA), 133n3
Conflict management problem as hindrance to health, 110–11
Constant demand on clergy as hindrance to health, 81–82
Contemplation of habits of health, 60–61
Corruption of habits of health, 19–21, 33–35
Courage as acquired virtue, 70–71, 99–100, 125
Cycling, 134

De Anima (Aristotle), 40–41
Decrease of habits of health, 19–21, 33–35
Descartes, René, 44
DiClemente, Carlo, 7, 54, 59, 61–62
Diet, 4, 8, 56–57, 91–92, 99–100, 120
Disability
  dealing with, 51–53
  teleology and, 71–73
Disease
  dealing with, 51–53
  teleology and, 71–73
Drinking, 69
Dualism, 39n1, 40–42, 50, 85–86
Duke Divinity School, 79, 86
Duke Endowment, 79
Duke University Institutional Review Board, 105n11

Ecclesial communities, 77–79
  health statistics among, 78
  stress among, 77n1
Eidos (form), 40
Embodied passion, 50–51
Emotion, passion for health compared, 47nn2–3
Ends of habits of health, 64–73

acquired virtues, 66–71 (*See also* Acquired virtues)
Aristotle on, 12–16
eudaimonia (living well in accordance with virtue) as, 65
God as, 22–23
overview, 7, 37–38, 64, 73
theological virtues, 65–66 (*see also* Theological virtues)
virtuous life as, 65–71
Energeia (activity), 15
Ensouled passion, 50–51
Entelechy (body), 40
Entitative habits, 44–46
Eucharist, 133–34
Eudaimonia (living well in accordance with virtue)
  Aristotle on, 11, 15–16
  as end of habits of health, 65
  habits of health, resulting from, 132
  operative habits and, 44
Exercise, 91–92, 95–96, 99, 120. *See also* Running

Faith as theological virtue, 65
Field work, health challenges for, 108–9
Flourishing, increase in, 92–93
Food. *See* Diet
Friendship, 133

Gnosticism, 85–86
Goals of habits of health. *See* Ends of habits of health
God
  as end of habits of health, 22–23
  kingdom of, 116–17
  in suffering, 115–16
  theoria (focus on God), 14–16
Goodness, health and, 88
"Good shepherds," health and, 87
Grace, habits of health as infused by, 21–22, 37

Habits of health
  actions of, 54–63 (*see also* Actions of habits of health)

149

Subject Index

agency of habit, action as, 18–19, 32–33
Aquinas on, 17–38 (*see also* Aquinas, Thomas (Saint)—on habits of health)
Aristotle on, 9–16 (*see also* Aristotle—on habits of health)
charity, impact on, 134–36
church, impact on, 132–134
Clergy Health Initiative and, 90–91
ends of, 64–73 (*see also* Ends of habits of health)
entitative habits and body, 44–46
God as end of, 22–23
grace, as infused by, 21–22, 37
increase, decrease or corruption of, 19–21, 33–35
instinct contrasted, 19n10, 57n17
as lasting quality, 18, 31–32
as ongoing journey, 94–95
operative habits and soul, 43–44
overview, 5–8, 31
repetition of, 19, 33
routine compared, 17n2
science as, 18n9
in secular programs, 36n46
transformation resulting from, 131–32
virtue, disposing toward, 21, 35–36
Word Made Flesh and, 124
Hadewijch, 135
Health
Aquinas on, 24–31 (*see also* Aquinas, Thomas (Saint)—on health)
as habit, 26–27
habits of (*See* Habits of health)
holistic approach to, 39–46 (*see also* Holistic approach to health)
idol, not deemed, 29
passion for, 47–53 (*see also* Passion for health)
salvation, not deemed, 28–29
as status, 25–26
summum bonum (greatest good), not deemed, 29
WHO definition of, 30–31
Heuertz, Phileena, 113–14
Hindrances to health
administrative burdens, 111
appointment system as, 84–85
catechesis in health, lack of, 81
conflict management problem, 110–11
constant demand on clergy, 81–82
institutional barriers, 110–11
"martyrdom" problem, 82–83
negative or absent teachings about health, 105–7
pastoral leadership, lack of, 113
"people pleaser" problem, 84
sacrifice expectation, 107–8
"Savior complex," 82–83
"sink or swim" culture, 110, 125
theological hindrances, 85–86
time management problem, 81–82
vision, uncertainty regarding, 111–12
workaholism, 109
Holistic anthropology, 40–42
Holistic approach to health, 39–46
Aquinas on, 40–42
Clergy Health Initiative and, 89
entitative habits and body, 44–46
holistic anthropology, 40–42
operative habits and soul, 43–44
overview, 7, 39
Holy Spirit, 65, 88, 97, 132
Homer, 9
Honoring the Body (Paulsell), 96
Hope as theological virtue, 65

Idol, health not deemed, 29
Increase of habits of health, 19–21, 33–35
Instinct, habits of health contrasted, 19n1, 57n17
Institutional barriers to health, 110–11
Intellect, habits of health and, 55n1
Interview questions
Clergy Health Initiative, 138–139
Word Made Flesh, 137–138

Jesus
generally, 103, 114, 118, 126, 132, 135
Aquinas on, 6, 16, 21, 23

Subject Index

death and, 52, 72
Eucharist, 133–34
holism and, 85
on love, 91
"martyrdom" and, 82–83
Resurrection, 88n20
salvation and, 28
"Savior complex" and, 82–83
John Paul II (Pope), 72, 135
Justice as acquired virtue, 68–69, 125

Keating, Thomas, 114–15
Kempe, Margorie, 135
Kingdom of God, 116–17

Lasting quality, habits of health as, 18, 31–32
Logos, 9n1
Love
  Jesus on, 91
  as theological virtue, 66
Luther, Martin, 98

Maintenance of habits of health, 62–63
"Martyrdom" problem as hindrance to health, 82–83, 134–36
Metaphysics (Aristotle), 26
Missionaries, health challenges for, 108–9
Multiple sclerosis, 3–5

Nicomachean Ethics (Aristotle), 12
Nominalism, 39n1
Norcross, John C., 7, 54, 59, 61–62
North Carolina Conference of the United Methodist Church, 79

Ongoing journey, habits of health as, 94–95
Operative habits, 43–44

Pagans, virtue and, 64n1, 66nn11–12
Passion for health, 47–53
  disability, dealing with, 51–53
  embodied passion, 50–51
  emotion compared, 47nn2–3
  ensouled passion, 50–51
  overview, 7, 47–48

  sickness, dealing with, 51–53
  virtue and, 48–49
Pastoral leadership, lack of as hindrance to health, 113
Paul (Saint), 88
Paulsell, Stephanie, 96
"People pleaser" problem as hindrance to health, 84
Potesis (production), 13–15
Praxis (action), 15–16
Precontemplation of habits of health, 60
Preparation for habits of health, 61
Prima Secundae (Aquinas), 17, 135, 139
Primitive Physic (Wesley), 89
Prochaska, James, 7, 54, 59, 61–62
Prudence as acquired virtue, 67–68, 99, 124
Psychological stages of change, 58–63
  action, 61–62
  contemplation, 60–61
  maintenance, 62–63
  precontemplation, 60
  preparation, 61
Purpose of habits of health. *See* Ends of habits of health

Reason, habits of health and, 56–57
Relationship between theology and health, 97–98
Repetition of habits of health, 19, 33
Res cognitans (mental substance), 41, 44
Res estensa (corporeal substance), 41
Resurrection, 88n20
"Rhythm of life," health and, 119–20
Routine, habit compared, 17n2
Running
  generally, 32n31
  as action of habits of health, 54, 59–63
  courage and, 70–71
  as habit of health, 24, 31–38
  "hitting the wall," 71n38
  justice and, 68–69
  overview, 4, 7, 24
  prudence and, 67–68

151

Subject Index

temperance and, 69–70

Sacrifice expectation as hindrance to health, 107–8
Saint Augustine, 18
St. Benedict's Monastery, 114
Saint Paul, 88
Saint Thomas Aquinas. *See* Aquinas, Thomas (Saint)
Salvation, health not deemed, 28–29
Salvifici Doloris (John Paul II), 72
"Savior complex" as hindrance to health, 82–83
Schwengel, Dr., 3–4
Science as habit, 18n9
Secundae Secundae (Aquinas), 133
Self-improvement programs, 73n46, 132n2
Sex, 69
Shuman, Joel, 133
Sickness
  dealing with, 51–53
  teleology and, 71–73
Sin, role in health, 8n5, 73n46
"Sink or swim" culture as hindrance to health, 110, 125
Socrates, 9
Sorrow, 50
Status, health as, 25–26
Stewardship, health and, 87
Storey, Peter, 100
Struggle for health. *See* Passion for health
Study methodology
  Clergy Health Initiative, 80–81
  Word Made Flesh, 104–5
Suffering, presence of God in, 115–16
Summa Theologiae (Aquinas), 6, 17, 94, 139
Summun bonum (greatest good), health not deemed, 29
Supplements, 4–5
"Sustainability," health and, 119–20

Techne (craft), 13–14
Telos. *See* Ends of habits of health
Temperance as acquired virtue, 69–70, 99, 124

Temple, body as, 88
Theological hindrances to health, 85–86
Theological virtues, 65–66
  charity, 65–66
  faith, 65
  hope, 65
  love, 66
  relationship to acquired virtues, 65n9
Theoria (focus on God), 14–16
Therese of Liseaux, 28
Thomas Aquinas (Saint). *See* Aquinas, Thomas (Saint)
Time management problem as hindrance to health, 81–82
Treatise on Habit (Aquinas), 24, 72
"True self," learning, 114–15
24/7 mentality, 134–36

Ultimate science, 14–16
United Methodist Church
  generally, 135
  appointment system, 84–85
  Clergy Health Initiative, 77–101 (*see also* Clergy Health Initiative)
  holism and, 89
  needs to address, 100–101

Virtue
  acquired virtues, 66–71 (*see also* Acquired virtues)
  Aquinas on, 21, 35–36
  Aristotle on, 10–11
  eudaimonia (living well in accordance with virtue) (*see Eudaimonia* (living well in accordance with virtue))
  habits of health as disposing toward, 21, 35–36
  pagans and, 64n1, 66nn11–12
  passion for health and, 48–49
  theological virtues, 65–66 (*see also* Theological virtues)
Virtuous life as end of habits of health, 65–71
Vitamins, 4–5

Subject Index

Wadell, Paul, 131–32
Wellbeing, theology of, 114–17
Wesley, John, 89–90, 98–99, 135, 138–39
Western North Carolina Conference of the United Methodist Church, 79
Will, habits of health and, 55–56
Word Made Flesh, 102–29
  ability to change and adapt, 127
  administrative burdens, health and, 111
  Clergy Health Initiative compared, 126–28
  conflict management problem as hindrance to health, 110–11
  field work, health challenges for, 108–9
  habits of health and, 124
  health resources, increase in, 121–22
  hindrances to health, 105–13
  institutional barriers to health in, 110–11
  institutional changes in, 120–23, 126–27
  institutional support in, 127
  interview questions, 137–38
  kingdom of God and, 116–17
  missionaries, health challenges for, 108–9
  needs to address, 125
  negative or absent teachings about health in, 105–7
  new habits adopted by, 117–20
  openness to transformation, 122–23
  overview, 7–8, 78–79, 102–4, 125–26, 129
  pastoral leadership, lack of, 113
  results of study, 123–25
  "rhythm of life," health and, 119–20
  sacrifice expectation as hindrance to health, 107–8
  "sink or swim" culture as hindrance to health, 110, 125
  spiritual practices, changes in, 117–19
  study methodology, 104–5
  suffering, presence of God in, 115–16
  "sustainability," health and, 119–20
  theological foundation of health in, 123
  theological training in, 128
  transformation resulting from habits of health, 131–32
  "true self," learning, 114–15
  vision of, uncertainty regarding, 111–12
  wellbeing, theology of, 114–17
  workaholism as hindrance to health, 109
Workaholism as hindrance to health, 109
World Health Organization (WHO) definition of health, 30–31

Yoga, 134

153

Names Index

Angela of Foligno, 135
Aquinas, Thomas (Saint), 6–8, 6nn3–4, 8n5, 13, 16–33, 17n1, 18n3, 18nn5–9, 19nn10–12, 20nn14–21, 21nn22–23, 22nn26–27, 23n34, 24nn1–2, 25nn3–8, 26n12, 26nn9–10, 27nn13–14, 28nn16–17, 29n23, 31nn29–30, 32n32, 33nn34–35, 33nn37–38, 34nn39–41, 35nn42–45, 36–50, 37n47, 40nn5–8, 41n9, 41n11, 42nn12–13, 43nn14–17, 44nn18–22, 45nn23–28, 46nn29–32, 47nn2–3, 48nn7–8, 49n14, 50n19, 50n21, 51nn22–23, 52n29, 53–56, 55nn1–4, 56n7, 56nn9–10, 57nn11–15, 58, 58nn19–22, 59nn23–25, 60–63, 64n1, 65–66, 65n2, 65nn8–9, 66nn10–11, 67n19, 67nn15–17, 68–69, 68nn22–24, 70n37, 70nn34–35, 72–73, 72n40, 73n46, 78–80, 79n5, 81n14, 82, 84, 90–93, 95, 97–99, 101, 105n11, 113, 114n13, 115n15, 124–25, 124n18, 129, 131–33, 133n5, 139
Aristotle, 7, 9–26, 9n2, 10nn3–5, 10nn8–9, 11n10, 11nn13–14, 12nn15–19, 13n21, 14n25, 14n27, 15nn29–31, 18n6, 18n9, 19n11, 20n14, 21n23, 25n8, 26n12, 27nn13–14, 29, 32, 32nn32–33, 38, 40, 42n13, 43n15, 45, 45n28, 46n29, 47n1, 47n3, 48n8, 57n13, 57n15, 63, 68–69, 131, 133, 133n4

Augustine (Saint), 18, 18n7

Barth, Karl, 27n15, 48n9, 51–52, 51n24, 52nn25–28, 71n39, 73n44, 92, 92n23, 129, 129n19, 135
Bauerschmidt, Frederick Christian, 28n17, 133n5
Bell, Catherine, 134n7
Berry, Wendell, 133–34, 133n3, 134n8
Brown, Stephen F., 65n5
Brumberg, Joan Jacobs, 30n28

Cates, Diana Fritz, 10nn7–8, 11n11, 15n30, 18n4, 47n1, 49n12, 50n20
Chandler, E. N., 77n3
Charmaz, K., 80n13
Conrad, Peter, 29n24
Curless, Melanie, 104n8, 108n12

Descartes, René, 44
Dewey, John, 59n23
DiClemente, Carlo, 7, 54, 59, 59n23, 59n25, 60nn26–27, 61–62, 61nn28–29, 62n30
Dillon, Dana, 40n5, 41n10
Dionysius, 21n22
Dunnington, Kent, 17nn1–2, 20n21, 49n11, 56n8, 57nn16–17, 58n18
Dwelle, T.L., 102n2

Empedodes, 9n1
Evans, Abigail Rian, 28n19

Francis, L. J., 77n2

Galen, 25n8

155

Names Index

Gallagher, David M., 55n5, 56n6
Griffith, R. Marie, 36n46, 73n46, 123n17

Hadewijch, 73n45, 135
Haley, Tara, 104n8, 108n12
Hall, Amy Laura, 65n9
Heuertz, Phileena, 103n5, 103n7, 104n8, 108n12, 113–14
Holifield, E., 138n1
Homer, 9
Huetter, Reinhard, 43n14
Hughes, Melanie Dobson, 89n21
Hughes, W. D., 21n22, 44n18

Iverson-Gilbert, J., 77n1

James, William, 59n23
Jesus, 6, 16, 21, 23, 28, 52, 72, 82–83, 85, 88n20, 91, 103, 114, 118, 126, 132–35
John of the Cross, 73n45
John Paul II (Pope), 72, 72nn41–43, 135

Keating, Thomas, 114–15, 114n14
Kempe, Margorie, 135
Kenny, Anthony, 42n12, 43n16, 44n18, 50n21
Kent, Bonnie, 10n6, 22n26, 28n18, 29n20, 57n15, 65n8
Klima, Gyula, 40n4
Klubertanz, George, 6n2, 17n2, 46n31, 59n23
Knight, Kelvin, 13n21, 14n27, 14nn23–24, 15n28, 16n32

Lange, W. R., 102n1
Lee, C., 77n1
Lombard, Peter, 22n26
Luther, Martin, 98, 98n24

MacIntyre, Alastair, 10n8, 11n12
Maddox, Randy, 89n22, 138n1
Mattison, William, 21n25, 33n36, 47n3, 67n17, 67nn20–21, 68n25, 68n27, 70nn34–35
McKenny, Gerald, 6n1, 13n22, 30n26

Meisenhelder, J. B., 77n3
Miner, Robert, 47n3, 49n14, 50n16, 50n19

Norcross, John C., 7, 54, 59, 59n23, 59n25, 60nn26–27, 61–62, 61nn28–29, 62n30
Nussbaum, Martha, 9n1, 14n26

Oesterle, John A., 18n9, 44n21
Overmyer, Sheryl, 64n1, 65n9, 66n12, 66n14

Paul (Saint), 88
Paulsell, Stephanie, 96, 123n17
Pierce, Charles, 59n23
Plato, 9n1, 14n27
Pope, Stephen, 49n13, 65nn3–4, 65nn6–8, 69n29, 70nn36–37
Porter, Roy, 11n14, 25n8
Prochaska, James, 7, 54, 59, 59n23, 59n25, 60nn26–27, 61–62, 61nn28–29, 62n30
Proeschold-Bell, Rae Jean, 77n1, 80n13
Putnam, Ruth Anna, 17n2

Rowatt, W., 77n1

Schwengel, Dr., 3–4
Shuman, Joel, 6n1, 17n2, 22n31, 29n22, 30n27, 39n2, 133, 133n6, 134n7
Socrates, 9, 9n1
Storey, Peter, 100
Swinton, John, 123n17

Therese of Liseaux, 28
Titus, Craig Steven, 49n10
Torrell, Jean-Pierre, 8n5, 22n29, 40n3, 66n14, 67n18, 73n46
Turton, D. W., 77n2

Verhey, Allen, 29n21

Wadell, Paul, 19n13, 22n28, 22n30, 23nn32–33, 47n4, 48nn5–7, 49n15, 55n4, 58n22, 66nn13–14,

Names Index

69nn30–33, 79n5, 129n20, 131–32, 132n1
Wesley, John, 89–90, 89n21, 98–99, 135, 138–39, 138n1
West, Silas, 103nn6–7

White, Kevin, 49n14, 50nn16–18
Wieland, George, 64n1

www.ingramcontent.com/pod-product-compliance
Lightning Source LLC
Chambersburg PA
CBHW050820160426
43192CB00010B/1839